THE KIDNEY WARRIORS

A Clan That Possesses Extraordinary Power to Overcome Challenges

Vasundhara Raghavan

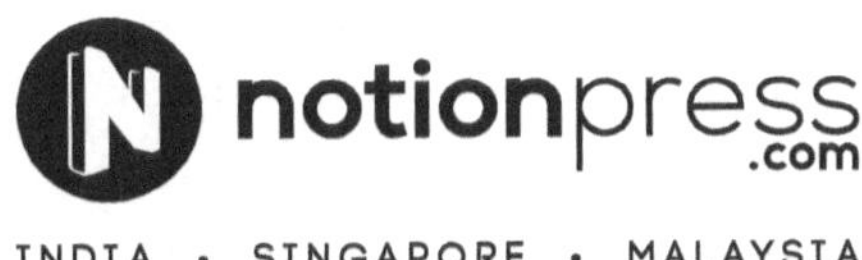

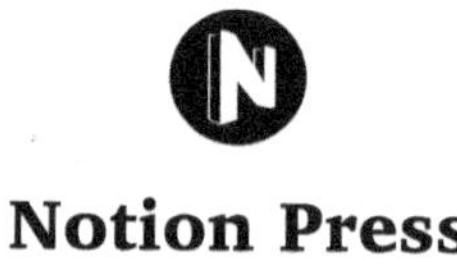

Notion Press

Old No. 38, New No. 6
McNichols Road, Chetpet
Chennai - 600 031

First Published by Notion Press 2018
Copyright © Vasundhara Raghavan 2018
All Rights Reserved.

ISBN 978-1-64249-710-6

Acceptance and management of the disease are aspects beyond a common man's understanding.

Saluting them for their quiet endurance.

"What is man, when you come to think upon him, but a minutely set, ingenious machine for turning with infinite artfulness, the red wine of Shiraz into urine?"

Isak Dinesen, Danish author (1885-1962)

CONTENTS

PART -1

PART – 2

INTRODUCTION

I was finishing up my final round of shopping before Diwali and the rush in the mall was unimaginable. Suddenly, I felt annoyed by a strong stench, which is so familiar in our routine lives. "Oh! Can we never escape this smell outside a public toilet?" As much as this irked me, I continued to actively speculate about it.

"Urine" has always been a topic that people avoid discussing as it's considered to be too personal. Our sense of propriety tells us that it's unsophisticated to openly talk about such things. But, at some point, this subject needs exploring in order to understand its relevance in our lives. The odour provokes instant disgust, and due to its high waste content, there's a scientific reason behind condemning it to the darkest recesses of our households, where toilets are generally situated.

Urine's other close association is with the bladder, an organ that gets randomly referred to when it's full; an expression used when nothing but the urge to urinate occupies a person's mind. At that moment, one can only think about reaching the closest toilet!

It suddenly dawned on me that **kidneys, *the factory*** that manufactures urine, is never in any of our thoughts. Most people are not aware of the methodical segregation done by the kidneys – a process through which it removes excess fluid and electrolytes while accurately retaining the amount potentially needed for the body's functioning. Ignorance is bliss till *the factory's* machinery breaks down and the body is flooded with excess waste and fluid.

This breakdown, unfortunately, is life-threatening. It is a life-long struggle to try to set our kidneys right. It requires a humungous and painstaking effort, full of endless experiments, to get it perfect. Though most of us are lucky to have 2 kidneys, both get compromised when *the factory* shuts down. Cost determines our survival plan, making demarcation of the economically weaker section more visible. The person would then face extremely troubled times with constant worry on their minds: "Will I be?" or "Will I not be?"

Ironically, urine, which was a topic we never discussed, becomes the focus of our conversations. One then begins to understand how a diseased kidney can change our lives and future. It's a permanent change that leaves scars on one's psyche.

If you were to survey people on what they think about kidney failure, the instinctive response would probably be dialysis and transplant. There's no pause to wonder if the complex disease that challenges people, as well as the attending physicians, has been adequately described. Then, almost as an afterthought, they will come up with another important connection: the kidney organ trade in India. In one stroke, the person and the doctor are doomed to disrepute. Sadly, this also means that the focus has shifted away from the person with the kidney disease!

From the time a person receives news of the 'kidney failure', life comes to a full stop. People around may offer counsel, but life is tough with the disease. There is a lot of loneliness and insecurity. The economic burden of survival is very high for all classes of the society; a patient in the middle-income group spends nearly 50% of their monthly income on treatment and medications. Living on dialysis is a huge financial strain. Seeking a kidney transplant is riddled with problems like finding a donor. Costs are high at all stages of the disease.

The young may stop their education and people in the age group of 25 to 35 years either lose their jobs or voluntarily quit thinking life is at its end. People lose the power to think and execute a survival plan. In social circles, there's a tendency to maintain a distance from kidney patients. The fear of being approached for a kidney or financial help creates a wedge in relationships.

The world has to learn and understand that kidney disease can happen to anyone. It is beyond anyone's control. Sometimes it's genetic, sometimes congenital and very often, it's beyond their understanding that **diabetes** and **hypertension** could drive them to kidney disease. Both diabetes and hypertension are the largest and most aggressive reasons for growth of the disease. Drug-induced cases are prominent as well. Environmental factors also contribute to gradual dents in people's health and make them more susceptible to the disease.

Real concern for human lives needs to replace doubt and judgement of people purely on hearsay. Today, if a 25-year-old faces kidney failure, which is not congenital or genetic, the world needs to worry and ask questions such as *"Why are young people facing such a life-threatening health disease?"*

Ever imagined a person's physical condition in the advanced stages of the disease? One may try to visualise it. Imagine the consequence of all toilets being shut down for a whole day. Any normal person would be uncomfortable if he's not able to urinate! Every hour of holding it in will make the person irritable and increase his discomfort. For a person with chronic kidney disease, the urge to urinate may be missing but carrying the fluid load with toxins makes them uncomfortable. But they play the greatest game of "charades" as they remain smiling as if they are as normal as others around them.

This book is very special to me. It has stories of people from across several states in India. Our attempt has been to make the reader privy to details about kidney disease and understand the raw emotions of a person standing in a dangerous crevice, uncertain about survival. There will be empathy, shock and tremors when one reads about the affronts and humiliation these patients have faced!

You will feel sadness as well as pride to see them rise after a fall and appreciate the ascent to glory that these people have achieved despite being on dialysis. Each story has the same thread of experience, but each person walks out of a different household. Social aspects have added flavour to the complexity of their lives.

This book is for readers to understand and arrive at conclusions with an honest heart; not to believe that you can judge another person on how he/she has conducted his/her life, but to imagine how you would survive if you were in their shoes. At different crossroads, their decisions largely depended on their family background and the environment they lived in. They can't be judged from a distance from the comfort of a secure home. That's the stark truth.

You will hopefully awaken to see what causes concerns. It will be clear that chronic kidney disease is not merely a physical condition. It is also an emotional battle for patients; you can clearly see they are playing in an unequal battleground among able-bodied people with similar income and struggling to make ends meet because huge medical bills, which are not covered by any insurance, need to be handled through their hard work.

If one is horrified at the prospect of a divorce, then welcome to this world. Apart from battling the disease, the patient is often left alone to pick up the shreds of a broken home and to handle the disease as well as manage it on a single or no income. Think of a kid born to a mother who dies of kidney disease and whose father has forsaken him. Without the umbrella of a secure household, how would that child, also suffering from the disease, lead a normal life, on par with people receiving love from parents?

The stories in this book are not inspired from movie scripts. They are as true as the bright, burning sun on the horizon and the blueness of the water in the ocean. Sharing their stories is a bold step for these people. They understand how the lack of awareness, even among people close to them, has destroyed the edifice of strong relationships. They are willing to lead by example.

Every single one of them will strongly vouch for the fact that this part of their life has been more heartbreaking than any other challenge they've experienced; it's more mentally exhausting than pangs of loneliness caused by loving partners drifting away or seeing their career-related dreams shatter.

Worldwide, the number of people suffering from kidney diseases is rising, and there's concern for the future. There's no cure in sight for some very rare diseases. Medicines are exorbitantly priced and are not within reach of even the higher income groups in India as well as in first world countries. Better organ donation laws, medical insurance schemes and guaranteed employment opportunities will go a long way in improving the lives of people who have fought bravely against these diseases.

I see them as people who are recognisable due to their grit. They have a zest for life, making an impactful statement that life is but for living. These are the stories of only a handful of people, but one can imagine there are many more who have vowed to survive.

All of them truly belong to the tribe – The Kidney Warriors.

Vasundhara Raghavan

Author

PART – 1

HEARTWARMING STORIES BASED ON FACTS AND INCIDENTS OF THEIR LIFE

GOOD STRATEGIC PLAN TO SURVIVE

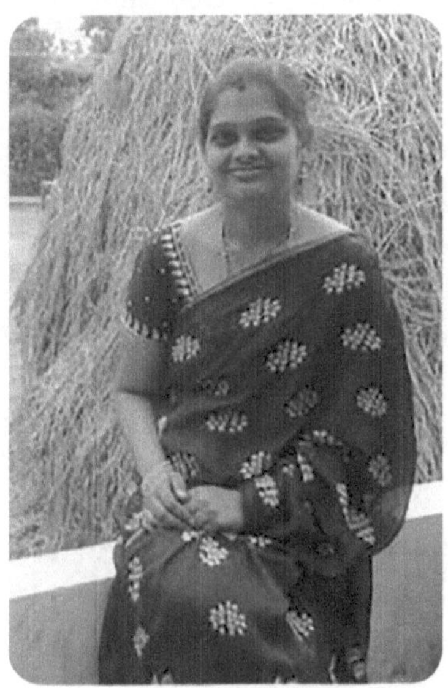

Nephrotic Syndrome

When I look back on my childhood, sometimes I wonder *how did so much happen to me that I never quite understood it at that time?* But when I was detected with kidney failure, I could suddenly connect the dots of times of greatest confusion and those of extreme discomfort.

One has to simply reflect on how these difficult situations in a girl child's life could have completely destroyed her confidence.

But, amazingly, I survived.

For my family, it meant many financial hurdles. They had to find money to save me.

But they managed to raise funds and I survived.

Today, as a married lady, I stand confident and happy because my husband never judged me. He understood and accepted me as I am. His strong support has been comforting, particularly because he never considered that my health condition was due to any fault of mine. It was all as God had willed.

I never allow myself to forget those early years of childhood spent in the district of Gudivada, situated some 40 to 50 km away from Vijayawada. Episodes of bed-wetting had troubled me till I was in class 9. It upset my mother so much that I could feel nothing but disappointment thinking I had hurt her terribly. Not willing to ignore it, my parents consulted a few doctors, but we were assured that it would get resolved.

And then one day, to my amazement, it stopped. Suddenly, life changed so dramatically. I found life so wonderful. I truly enjoyed this spell of happiness to its fullest. Life seemed so exciting. It seemed as if my life's path had changed overnight and I could think of nothing but the pleasures of life.

Without any forewarning, some problems surfaced. I still remember the incident very vividly. I started experiencing some uneasiness just before my 10th standard exams. It soon led to nausea and I vomited very frequently. We met a general physician who prescribed medicines to stop the nausea. But at that time, no other tests were conducted. I recall how I was down with a fever so often.

I joined a university to further my education, which meant living in a hostel. One day, while walking up the hostel's stairs, I fell and rolled down the steps. Though there was no injury at that time, I noticed that a swelling had developed in my legs.

Somehow, I believed it was due to the fall. When we visited a doctor, he examined it and nodding his head, he said, "This is oedema; water has accumulated in the body. I suggest you get some tests done."

The urine analysis report identified the problem. There was the presence of albumin in the urine.

In a confused state of mind, my family made an appointment with a nephrologist. A biopsy was done, and it was concluded that I was suffering from Nephrotic Syndrome. The doctor was kind enough to assure us positively, saying there was hope for survival with a kidney transplant.

As a young lady, I was tremendously shocked!

"What is all this?" I asked, devastated. "Why does everything pile up like this?"

Amma tried to console me and I noticed how disturbed *Appa* was to see me sad and heartbroken. He sat, fingers knotted, trembling and his eyes shone with unshed tears. He had always called me 'my princess!' But now, as much as I felt shattered, he was reeling under the doctor's verdict: a kidney failure.

Those were the toughest days of our lives. *Appa* would search through files to look for some documents and take down extensive notes. He would go to the hospital to find out more details about the transplant. Sometimes he would talk about it as if he were continuing an old conversation.

I always saw a lot of concern in his eyes. At times, I could read in them, "We will fight it, don't worry." But on other days, *Appa* would get depressed.

So, I went back to live with them, forgetting my education. Lots of discussion about the cost of transplant took place on a daily basis. *Appa* would enquire about kidney transplants from people who had got it done. I would hear my parents talk in whispers at night. *Amma* would say, "How can we do the transplant? You are saying it will cost about Rs 3.5 lakhs?"

Appa's voice would shake, "We have to find the money somehow. Sell the land, maybe?"

Somehow, it seemed as though most decisions were made during the quiet of the night. But finally, we managed to find funds and the transplant surgery was done.

What Exactly Made It Possible?

The first aspect that paved the path for survival was acceptance. This is a great word, but it has a very deep meaning; to learn to 'accept' takes time and is a long process. My family learnt it well as each problem surfaced and we found the right formula to overcome it.

During the process of accepting, *Appa* had started planning and he had an action plan. He began making progress in 2 directions: Arranging for the tests in the hospitals with my mother as the donor and looking for a buyer for our agricultural land. It was a small patch and his only security for old age and the future. At that point, nothing seemed to matter except selling the land and using all the proceeds for my surgery and treatments.

Appa only thought about keeping me alive.

Today, after 14 years with the new kidney, my husband plays a protective role. He is a pillar of support in ensuring that my health is always well-maintained. With so many sacrifices, I hope my life will always be steady.

Indu Priya
Dialysis: **2 months**
Transplant: **14 years**

MY PERSISTENCE BENEFITED ME

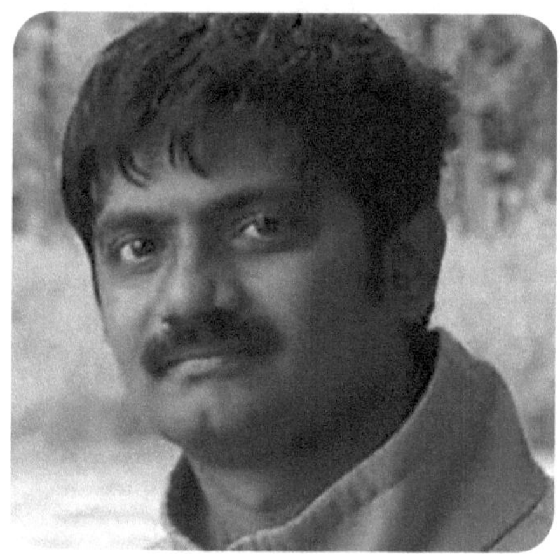

Rare disease: Alport syndrome

In my early years, I was diagnosed with hearing loss in both ears. Then, it seemed like my eyesight was poor as well. In 1992, out of desperation, I was shown to an ophthalmologist who waived it off as myopia. Challenged with only 2 partially working senses, I strove to work hard in school, as there was no other option in sight for me. Deep within, I did sometimes feel downcast, but I squashed the feeling and continued to sharpen my mind. I gained more knowledge and studied to the best of my capacity.

Suddenly, I was in the limelight. When graduating in Statistics, the university recognised my excellence in English by awarding me with 2 gold medals. My world changed. I felt upbeat. Partial eyesight and hearing were not even relevant anymore. I realised I had beaten the world. I simply felt happy and immensely proud. It was a period when I was blissfully unaware of anything that could possibly tip my apple cart.

Life moved on. I graduated with an MCA degree.

And then one day, in my 24th year, I was diagnosed with End-stage renal disease (ESRD). As knowledge seeped in and more questions crossed my mind, I investigated. I was diagnosed with Alport syndrome, a genetic disorder caused by the mutation in a gene. This disease is 3 pronged. It leads to sensorineural deafness, lens deformity in both eyes and kidney failure. The first defect was incurable; hearing aids helped me to some extent. The third defect, kidney failure, was life-threatening. Even as sadness filled my heart, I heard magical words of assurance from my uncle. "I want to donate my kidney," he said earnestly.

In a few months, the kidney transplant surgery was done. Settling with a new kidney changed many things. I was married to a nice lady, took a bank job and life saw an upswing with 2 daughters entering our home, one after the other. But at the same time, the second defect also seemed to be incurable. My wife and I went to many hospitals, only to return in despair. Finally, we came across a doctor who agreed to perform a difficult surgery. We were told there were risks involved in performing this surgery but we had complete faith in her. After 6 months, I had perfect vision.

Life with Alport syndrome is never easy. It occurred to me that throughout my schooling years I would never have reached this stage in life without such positive support from teachers. The school ensured that I was never treated differently, so my self-confidence was kept intact.

My wife was a rock of support when we went in search of treatment for my eye (lens) defect. She was steadfast in her quest to ensure that my eyes were treated.

Today, after 15 years, I am back on dialysis. I hope to get a kidney soon so that I can keep my spirits high. I have spent 17 years with Chronic Kidney Disease (CKD) and 35 years with hearing loss. I am still going strong and I intend to be so as long as I can.

Suri Gopichand
Andhra Pradesh

PS: This great warrior was a great intellectual, well read and a hard worker. Dialysis put a great strain on him. After almost 2 years on dialysis and a major surgery, he lost his fight. We salute him for being an active banker till his end.

FREEDOM WITH A KIDNEY TRANSPLANT

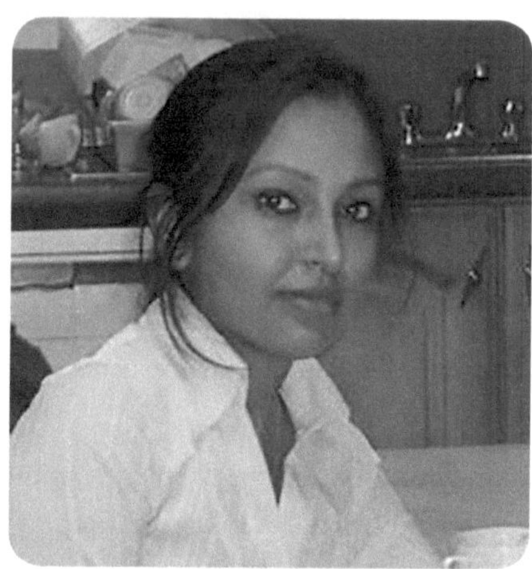

Hypertension

When I faced a life-threatening illness, I never expected to become a sturdy shock absorber. But today, after years of surviving many trials and tribulations, I'm a tough nut to crack.

I recall those times, now referred to as 'time before,' when life was filled with simple joys. One must just live by the moment. No worries or tensions crossed my path. It was all about office, friends and loads of fun. Then, a day arrived; it was a memorable day. I went for a medical check-up, and the doctor said thoughtfully, "There seems to be some problem. Traces of protein have been detected in the urine."

"Doctor, I am travelling to Ireland for corporate training. Can I travel?" I asked with some worry.

"It is not such a great problem. You can travel," he remarked casually. With great relief, I thanked him profusely and left his clinic after paying his fee. I was free to spread my wings and see my career take off. I had completed a Master's degree in mass communication, and professionally, I was satisfied with the overseas training as well as getting a managerial position. For a simple Bengali girl who belonged to a middle-class family living in Assam, working in Pune and going overseas for training was a big deal.

Then came 2009, which was monumental in every way!

I married another professional and life was so exciting and happy. After our wedding, we shifted to Delhi and later to Bangalore for work. Somehow, none of this city hopping really mattered to me. They were small changes, and I went with the flow. But when major changes surfaced, I experienced my life's greatest challenge.

One day, as I was getting ready to go to work, all of a sudden I felt breathless. I took a moment to think about this discomfort. *Should I skip work and take some rest?*

I decided to stay home. But my condition deteriorated in some time, so my husband rushed me to the hospital. Shockingly, my blood pressure (BP) was 220/120. The doctor quickly ordered some tests. The blood test revealed a high creatinine level at 5.6mg/dl. I was rushed to the ICU. My parents were summoned and we fell into a loop of visiting hospitals and doctors for further medical opinions. All the hospitals, as well as doctors, showed me the best way was to get a kidney transplant.

Kidney transplant meant we had to embark on a hunt for an eligible donor. On my own, I rejected my parents as prospective donors because they were aged and had medical issues; they were not suitable candidates for kidney donation.

My husband introduced me to an ayurvedic doctor. The medicines given by him brought down my creatinine to 2.2mg/dl in 5 months.

Before resuming work, I went to live with my parents at Silchar to recuperate. The few days of trying to collect my thoughts to get back some courage was the time I most needed to become more relaxed. But life changed very soon.

We received a call from my mother-in-law that left us shell-shocked. It was an outburst about how my husband's life was being affected by my ill health. The next few minutes were blurred. I remember I had collapsed with a thud. Many calls later, my mother murmured, "Your mother-in-law called. She is unhappy about your condition and is suggesting a divorce." It was an agonising time. Our peace was shattered.

Finally, my husband called me and said, "I think it is over. We must get a divorce." In my extremely weak state of mind, I spoke emotionally, "Why? Why do you want to give me a divorce?" He replied in anger, "You know why. Ask yourself." Even though I was breathing heavily, he spoke in an unfamiliar tone, "Your blood test had shown traces of protein and you concealed it from me, remember?" I cried, reasoned and pleaded innocence, but he was in no mood to listen. The drama continued. My pleading gave him a position of power.

He softened enough to say, "Yes, you can live with my second wife and me."

I was clueless about how to handle the 2 deep losses; losing a relationship that I had nurtured and seeing my life compromised by kidney failure were both life-changing. I felt threatened by the situations that entered my life together. My marriage had hit rock bottom and my family was deeply affected as their limited savings had been spent on my marriage. At no time did the disease become a second priority in my life. I was both physically and mentally bruised! I stayed away from everyone and I felt lost and defeated. There remained no joy in life. I was eating less, sleeping less and I stayed by myself in my room.

I tried to understand what had turned my loving husband against me. Every part of my body reacted with sorrow; my heart ached and my head reeled with worry. In this period, my health took a turn for the worse. I was rushed to the Intensive Care Unit (ICU) and was hooked to oxygen to keep me going.

This emergency changed everything. My family rallied around me. They responded very positively to me to bring me out of the throes of deep hurt and agony. My mother held my hands, and with her eyes shining with love, she said, "I'll give you my kidney, Lekha. Forget everything now. Only think of your health." Slowly, it dawned on me that my life was valuable to the people who mattered; people who loved and valued my existence.

A renowned Hyderabad doctor did my transplant surgery. Life changed miraculously. My self-confidence returned and I knew there was nothing better than moving ahead with life. I was finally in a condition to analyse my case better:

How is it possible that I never knew anything about kidney disease till 2012? Why did I not read the small details on the blood report and interpret it? Did the doctor ask me to come back for a follow-up, which I didn't pay heed to?

Without an answer to any of my musings, I gave up my search for theories.

I completed my first year of transplant and things seemed fine. But there was severe bleeding, so I was advised a pap smear. There were strong indications of cancer, so a colposcopy was done. My uterus was in very bad shape. To be doubly sure, a kidney biopsy was also done. Finally, to my relief, it was traced to be tuberculosis of the uterus. Within a year, I recovered completely with medications.

A few years back, the divorce came through, liberating me from an unworthy relationship.

Sometimes I think about my life-changing experiences. All of them brought about changes in me. I emerged as a stronger person who refuses to permit the shadows of a dark past ruin the present joys of life. There is relief in knowing I'm complete, intact and in possession of all the valuable things needed for a good life. I'm happy I don't have to crawl to find my identity and gain public acceptance. My family and friends rejoice in my being healthy, with my self-respect intact.

"You are my Warrior," she whispered. I looked up at my saviour, my loving mother, and knew I, indeed, had everything with me.

Chandralekha Das
Dialysis: 5 months
Transplant: 4 years

AN ATTITUDE TO SMILE THROUGH CKD

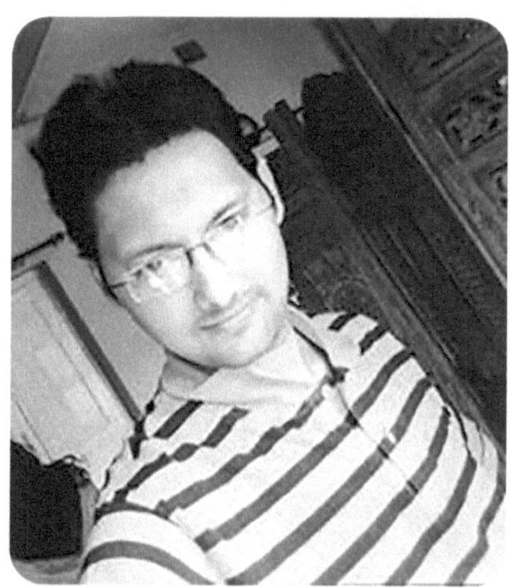

Hypertension

It always makes me laugh when people ask me, "You have such a serious disease, yet you're smiling? Are you not worried?"

Worried about what? My life will not change if I keep worrying and crying.

I was only 15 years old when I was detected with kidney failure. Papa asked the doctor, "How is that possible? Can it happen just like that? He's just a young boy. Please re-check and let us know."

The doctor saw me standing there. My innocent eyes were wondering and trying to understand more about my health. Taking a deep breath, he explained, "He has very high blood pressure and that has affected his kidneys. Please see this." He opened the report and showed us that the creatinine level was above the normal range.

After we came home, Papa and Mummy explained to me what kidney disease was. They assured me that there was nothing to worry about. They would take care of everything. I knew they meant every word of it. Papa and Mummy would do anything to save me.

Today, as I look back, I realise how much comfort their assurance had given me as a teenager. I cannot even imagine how I can be here, narrating it all!

From that day, I did everything that gave me joy. My mummy talked to me about diet and why I needed to make changes. I remember how it surprised me at that time, but I understood how important it was for the kidney and accepted her suggestions.

Very soon, a kidney transplant was scheduled. My mummy gave me her kidney. I became stronger and finished my degree in commerce.

I was a very active person. Though I didn't possess the talent to sing or dance, I spent lots of time with my cousins who were extremely talented. Gradually learning from them, I amused myself and kept myself happy. So, eventually, I concentrated on other aspects of life instead of just thinking about my health and disease.

In my 9th year post-transplant, my kidney showed signs of failing. Slowly, anxiety grew within me. I knew I had to face the disease again and felt insecure. *How would I get another transplant?*

I shared my fears and unhappy thoughts with Papa and Mummy. They would tell me stories of inspiration, of how Prophet Mohammad faced so many hardships and survived because of patience. They shared stories from religion about people who suffered day-to-day from many problems, about people who suffered because of poverty, cancer and other severe illnesses.

These stories showed me that I was not alone in my suffering. Millions of people had faced far greater problems with no economic means to overcome their problems. My mummy asked me to always look at people from lower-income households, how they managed with little food, no money for medicines and no proper house. They live with minimum support and few facilities. The suffering they experience in their day-to-day life is something no human being should ever have to deal with.

I noticed how Papa and Mummy managed to maintain peace and happiness in our family life without letting my disease make others miserable. So, I realised I should rise above my problems, without in any way allowing them to cast a shadow on anyone's life. I looked for opportunities to keep myself happy. Despite how difficult it was, I tried to keep all worries at bay.

Presently, I am back on dialysis. It is tough but I make every effort to remain happy. From a very early age, my parents inspired me to remain contented with life. Gradually I have developed an attitude to be happy whether with a transplanted kidney or while on dialysis.

I want every kidney patient who feels that the world has come to an end to know that we will live as long as we win over our problems. There is joy in overcoming problems with courage. More than that, it is all about learning to live life to the fullest.

Danish Haque
Dialysis: 3 years
Transplant: 9 years

GREATEST CHALLENGE OF POST-TRANSPLANT

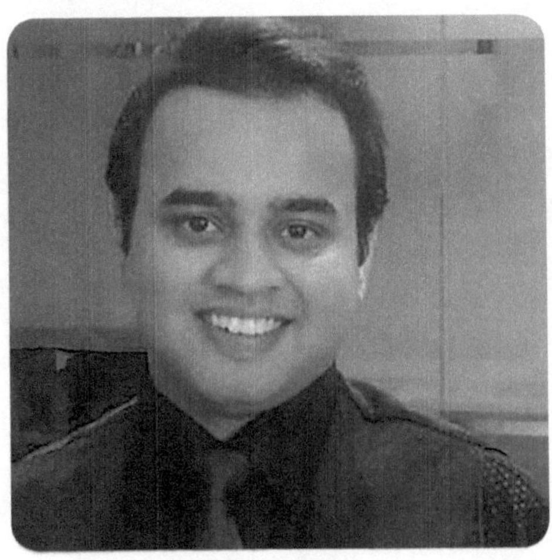

Hypertension

While living with a transplant means more freedom for me and I enjoy every moment of my life, I was disappointed that it comes with certain drawbacks too. I do not consider the side effects of the immunosuppressants to be a great cause for concern as they are a part and parcel of the renal replacement therapy. I have embraced the transplant process and the requisites for leading a good life in its entirety and learnt to understand as well as appreciate the reasoning behind it. I'm even happy to live with it.

My greatest challenge as a transplant recipient is how society often stigmatises my disease and reduces me to a mere diagnosis. I have faced discrimination at work and outside of work simply because I am living with a kidney transplant.

Given the fact transplant is an added financial burden for the recipient and his family, equal access to opportunities is often denied to the recipient. More understanding from people in industries to assist people in leading a normal life by providing some frill benefits not only helps people like me but makes society understand us as well. This is one aspect of my transplant which is perhaps most challenging for me. That too is not because of the disease but based on attitude.

Rishabh Bahl
Dialysis: some dialysis
Transplant: 3 years

SURVIVING A FATAL KIDNEY DISEASE

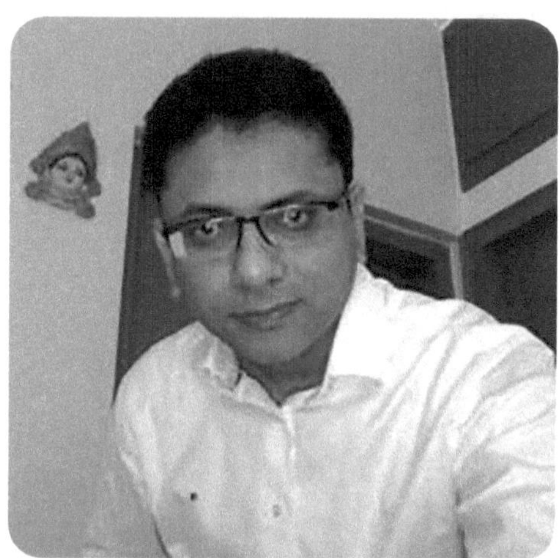

Autosomal Dominant Polycystic Kidney Disease

When and how one knows about their illness is not a time of their choosing. It happens at its calling. This is what I think now after going through the gamut of experiencing the life-threatening illness and walking back to my desk to write and publish my book, *Fight for life: My journey from a fatal disease to good health.*

Apart from everything narrated in the book and through pages where I have only made a subtle reference, I will give it full voice now. I feel that my fellow brethren need to know and feel the impact of my feelings.

During a pre-employment health check-up at the age of 23, I was in for a surprise. I got detected with Autosomal Dominant Polycystic Kidney Disease (ADPKD). The doctor began questioning about my family history with kidney disease and as a well-educated man, it set me thinking. Should I have ever speculated about it?

Years back, in 1983, my father died of kidney disease. His death meant dealing with a tragic loss, managing to live without him, creating new meanings to life and then life moved on. No one in my family looked down the corridor to see if the disease was loitering there, waiting to catch up with any of us! Unfortunately, my sister, who was a few years elder to me, became the second target of the disease even though she had a transplant after more than 2 years on dialysis. She was unlucky to have a post-transplant infection in the crucial first 3 months and then things went downhill from there as it led to other complications, resulting ultimately in her untimely death.

This disease grew slowly in me too, giving me a very tough time with excruciating pain. I tried many alternative treatments but all were in vain, and the inevitable did happen. Mine was a more complicated case than others as both my kidneys, which weighed almost 5 kgs, had to be removed in a surgery that almost took my life. I was on a ventilator and when I regained consciousness, I had to be on dialysis for some months before I could get a transplant. After the transplant, when I reflected on my time with the disease, many thoughts crossed my mind.

Many people went through similar experiences though one may say ADPKD is a very rare disease. In my case, the cysts took time to damage my kidneys. I had ample time to plan and summon courage. I had the fortune to work my way through a successful survival. I had a well-stimulated mind to process such complicated information and derive a conclusion that would benefit me. I also never let the disease in my family or me get me down and I stayed positive. How many people in India will have that window of opportunity?

I see many families with a member struggling with kidney disease. Many of them do not have the energy to look beyond what they are handling with the diseased person. I want to remind them that some kidney diseases are hereditary. If parents are affected, it will be beneficial for their kids to be tested; in the case of siblings, it is almost a 'must get done' as far as tests are concerned. The earlier one plans for a transplant the better. Even post-transplant, maintain discipline for a healthy life.

From experience, I can also say that this disease drains finances, so a little planning will help if detected early. And then, watch your progress closely. After all, survival is the best option.

Shantanu Saha
Dialysis: 4 months
Transplant: 6 years

SOME KIDNEY STONES ARE LIFE-THREATENING!

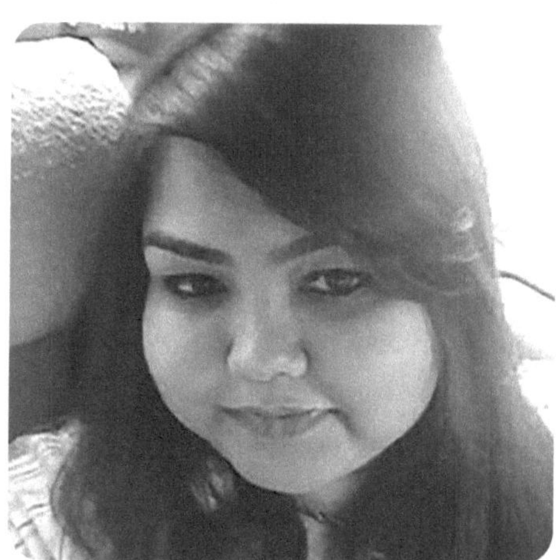

Primary Hyperoxaliuria type 2

My childhood was a fairytale; I had it all! Life was about being brought up with love and care by doting parents and a sibling who was a best friend. So, when I experienced an intense pain in the back, homeopathy was the chosen treatment due to my tender age. It was soft as well as gentle and gave me relief. Apart from those tiny, sweet homeopathic pills, I was advised an X-ray.

The kind doctor showed the X-ray image on a screen. I remember his finger pointing it out to my dad. "These are some stones that are forming here…" and he spoke in detail as I watched the men look very concerned. As I review my life in 2017, this is my first memory of kidney disease, at age 7.

Real and noticeable or things that a 13-year-old could comprehend happened when the back pain re-appeared. To avoid any invasive treatment, at our request, the doctor suggested Lithotripsy, which uses sound waves to break up large kidney stones into smaller pieces. Once broken down, the stones find it easier to pass through the bladder. Before beginning the treatment, I was warned that the right kidney would shrink due to the impact of the waves.

At this point, I also learnt that the stones were formed due to calcium oxalate stone formation. For the first time in my early teen years, I was being exposed to medical terms and treatments that were new even to my family members.

I sat there wondering and trying to understand what I was getting into. The doctor handed me a diet chart, gently explaining, "If you can maintain this diet, the stones will not form again."

I was advised to drink as much water as possible! I used to get very amused when I was introduced as the youngest stone former in the hospital.

Life seemed peaceful. I lived with a delusion of safety.

It came back with a bang, waking me up from my deep slumber. I was 23 years old and as unwelcome as it was, my blood test reports showed my creatinine was 4.5mg/dl. Tests revealed a massive stone in the left kidney. This led to hydronephrosis. My kidney was swollen and the passage for urine was blocked. Now I was in a position to decide, so I underwent a laser surgery to remove the stone. As advised, I went to a nephrologist to discuss the high creatinine. Miraculously, a month later, due to my strict medical compliance, my creatinine came down to 1.2.

I breathed, thinking a hurdle was crossed. But I did not rest. It was time to sort out this madness!

"I am extremely worried about this recurring stone formation! I suffer, get over it and start living, but then I come back to square one! Doctor, please help me unearth this to get to the root cause!" I discussed with the urologists, debated and pushed them to reason it out and to find me a conclusive solution to this traumatic experience. There were 3 more episodes that happened within a span of the next 2 years.

The tests were all clear, no specific ailment was found. It was down to 'predisposition to stone formation.'

Meanwhile, life took me to Bangalore, where I worked with an IT organisation. This was the best phase of my life, so upbeat and full of good friends. Life could not be better. I was able to manage work and health with a strict diet and regular check-ups. I was loving my life and living my dreams!

A sleeping snake will raise its hood; it seemed true for my kidney stones. It resurfaced in January 2013. By now, I could sense the symptoms. I was constantly weak and work didn't excite me anymore. On my parents' insistence, I shifted to Delhi. Some months later, on 6th November 2013, I suffered a uremic seizure. Further investigation revealed creatinine at 17 mg/dl. I had suffered kidney failure. That moment is forever etched in my mind.

It takes a few seconds for our life to change, I thought sadly.

After 2 months on dialysis, I underwent a transplant. There were numerous complications post-transplant. A biopsy of the graft revealed that there were numerous oxalate deposits. I underwent genetic testing at a Delhi hospital and then contacted the United States' famed Mayo clinic.

In last August, I was diagnosed with primary hyperoxaluria type 2. I was dealing with a classified rare disease that's caused by a genetic mutation. The only cure for this currently is a combined liver and kidney transplant. There's risk associated with such a transplant, with no great success rate. I was finally at peace, with the knowledge of what caused all this upheaval.

In a rare moment, I recalled a second opinion that came hours before my transplant. A nephrologist had suggested that my case was not appropriate for an isolated kidney transplant. At that time, our main nephrologist was confident that a kidney transplant was the best solution and at that point, we felt we couldn't walk out of the transplant. Such thoughts and memories make me wonder if a right decision can ever be made. After all, a coin does have 2 faces.

On 18ᵗʰ January 2017, I completed 3 years with the transplanted kidney. But the kidney has now developed nephrocalcinosis too. Over the years, fighting as hard as I have, my rising creatinine has also made no effort to relent. I went back on dialysis though the team of consulting doctors worked very hard to help me keep my kidney for as long as possible.

This time around though, I'm better prepared to handle the situation. Family and friends have been a great support through all of this.

I've learnt through the roughest patch of my life that though circumstances don't favour us always, we certainly can bank on ourselves. I'm contemplating a major career shift from a corporate job to being a baker to suit my lifestyle now. Nothing equals combining productivity with happiness.

Shruti Mukundan
Dialysis: 2 months
Transplant: 3 years
Dialysis again: 2 months till now

Life Revolves around Fighting Kidney Disease

Life was normal for us until the early morning of 6ᵗʰ November 2013. That is the day our fates changed forever. Shruti was diagnosed with kidney failure due to kidney stones and I felt like the whole world was crumbling down.

As a parent, I had built castles in the air about my daughter's future. She had a successful career and had infinite possibilities lying ahead of her. More than anything else, she is a loving and doting daughter. As much as I tried, I felt helpless and couldn't express how I felt. But I had to quickly rise to the occasion. My mind started racing for solutions. I was at a crossroads: **take a risk by getting a transplant or let her remain on dialysis?**

I wanted my daughter to regain good health quickly. With several opinions and going by her doctor's recommendation, my daughter got a kidney transplant.

Recently, when she was diagnosed with primary hyperoxaluria, I was devastated. My daughter's kidney failed because, for her disease, she required a dual organ transplant —kidney and liver.

Cut to 2017: After a failed kidney transplant, she's back on dialysis. I am very disappointed in many doctors who have treated Shruti since childhood. Had they diagnosed it earlier, adequate measures/medications could have been taken to avert kidney failure, quite possibly. Also, I admit my ignorance in never questioning doctors, but always taking things at face value as presented to me.

My only hope now is that if unrelated organ donation gets legalised, a lot of young lives would be saved. **My daughter has an option to live long only through a cadaver transplant.**

Lastly, I admire Shruti for her ability to withstand the calamities that overtook her life. Her 'everything is going to be alright' attitude is what keeps us going. She is our main reason to live!

P G Mukundan
Father

HOPE: A STRONG DRIVER

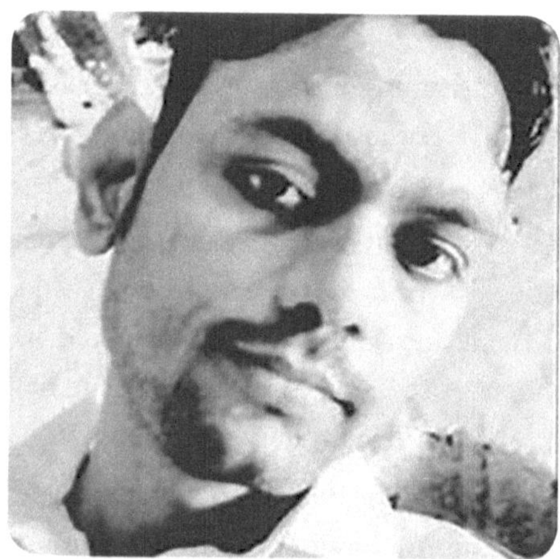

Membranoproliferative glomerulonephritis (MPGN)

At 14 years, I was sitting with a doctor and heard the words 'kidney disease.' These words were not in my dictionary. I sat looking at the doctor wonderingly. *What is he saying? Is he talking in Russian?* I continued to give him a blank stare. Surprisingly, my father's eyes widened in panic. He shook his head vigorously as if he would not accept it. Seeing my father, who was a mere farmer, look so scared as if he understood what was being said, I asked him, "Papaji, you know what the doctor is saying? How do you know?"

My father looked sad as he explained, "*Beta* (son), kidney disease is a very serious disease. You know, when I was young I went to a big university. There I studied Political Science and got a Master's degree. It is sad I had to go back to farming and could not educate you well enough. But now, Ved *beta*, you have to take care of your health as this disease can be dangerous."

Much later, when I grew older, I found out more about his education, but at an early age, I learnt about such a complex disease in great detail.

It all started with a very high fever. It turned out to be malaria. My condition was very serious and required admission into the city's government hospital for several months. After recovery, I tried leading a normal life, like all kids my age; attending school, playing cricket and cracking jokes to amuse myself. But the swelling in my face and legs made me feel strange and gave me a heavy feeling. Then, another fever took me back to my local doctor. Seeing my condition, he suspected it was a serious disease and sent me to the city hospital again. Tests were conducted - urine tests, blood test and a sonography.

That was the time these new words fell on my ears. The city doctor said, "Kidney disease," and my family was in a panic. The doctor comforted us saying, "We will start the treatment."

At that point, it not only meant going to the hospital every 15 days but we felt our pockets were emptied due to the high fees we had to pay. Little did we know then that a physician knows very little about kidney diseases; it is only a nephrologist who understands the disease! And so, I went, spent money and yet did not receive any real treatment.

In the meantime, I developed herpes zoster. This changed everything. The city doctor quickly referred me to the nephrology department at the All India Institute of Medical Sciences (AIIMS).

At AIIMS, a biopsy was done which revealed that I had membranoproliferative glomerulonephritis (MPGN).

The big words and the serious expression on the doctor's face just increased our fear levels. The doctor talked about how important it was to control my blood pressure with medicines and advised protein restriction. Once we left the hospital, the family huddled together and discussed what was to be done. Family and friends began advising us. We rushed from pillar to post, trying out homeopathy and ayurvedic medicines but gradually, I became sicker and reached end-stage renal failure.

By now, my mother had understood that to save me she would have to donate her kidney. In 2008, I received my 'new working kidney.' It was a happy time. People around me were curious and when I spoke, it was 'Greek and Latin' to them. Before I realised, 16 months had passed and my kidneys shut down again. MPGN had affected the kidneys. The disease had a tendency to reappear.

In the snakes and ladders game, I was at the bottom; at the starting point. The kidneys were not working anymore. My father had sold his farm to pay for my treatments and we hit an all-time low in morale – a weeping mother, a struggling father and a devastated me! With this kidney failure, we were truly a heartbroken family!

With kidney disease, one has to understand the importance of rising after a fall. And so, I went back to dialysis. Every now and then, small and big health issues still crop up. I have managed to overcome them with the help of people who love

me. They know and understand my health, as these problems are not new to them. Like me, they are also kidney warriors.

Ved Prakash Yadav
Dialysis -9 months
Transplant with mother as donor lasted: Few months
Dialysis – 7½ years

PS: As of January 2018: Ved received a cadaver transplant in August 2017. He is facing some issues and will soon be discharged from hospital very soon.

WILLPOWER BECAME MY LIFE'S SHIELD

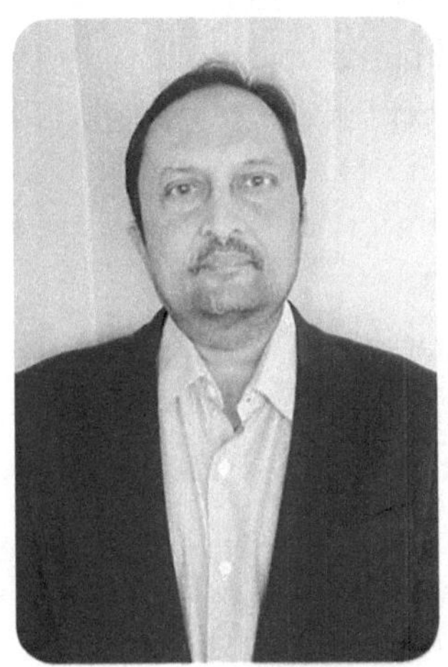

Hypertension

That day, 23rd November 1998, is still so fresh in memory, as it was the season of lights, colours, sweets and celebration in India.

I was woken up early that morning by sounds of twitters from the birds outside the window and sounds of the clatter of cups from the kitchen. As I opened my eyes, I felt my sight was blurred. I rubbed them clean, but it didn't help.

"Today is Diwali! There is so much excitement in the house, why are my eyes not able to see?" I questioned myself. My mind came up with a quick thought, *Am I losing my sight?*

I rushed to see an eye specialist. After a preliminary check-up, he suggested I meet a physician. My family doctor, who was a GP, checked my blood pressure. It was very high but there were no symptoms. He advised me to get a few tests done.

After a few hours, with my wife, I went to the doctor with the reports. I felt some uneasiness and knew it was my fear. To my utter surprise, the doctor pointed out my creatinine and said, "Such a high level means your kidneys are affected."

This was indeed very shocking news for us. We visited a nephrologist in Ahmadabad. The ultrasound showed that my kidneys had shrunk in size and the nephrologists explained that my kidneys were not working properly.

Fear drove us around the city to meet many doctors. We then went to Muljibhai Patel Urological Hospital, Nadiad to meet a renowned nephrologist. Though biopsy was advisable, my high BP made it impossible. So, we were clueless about the cause of the damage.

I saw this as the starting point of my battle for survival.

All this was so sudden; I broke down, felt shattered but in some part of my heart, hope was still alive. I decided to look for every option available for curing the disease. My search for medicines led me to homeopathy as well as Ayurveda and to McLeod Ganj, Dharamshala for treatments offered by His Holiness the Dalai Lama, from Buddhist practices.

One year was spent without any positive signs, but my confidence in recovery remained intact. Reports were stable and dialysis was not yet necessary.

Another date stands out: 26th January 2001.

Gujarat saw the most tragic earthquake. While the city was busy finding people squashed under debris, I faced one of my greatest challenges. My blood pressure shot up, my urea and potassium levels increased and I felt as if my life was falling apart. Emergency dialysis was started and I was now in the next stage of my fight for survival. Dialysis was recommended thrice a week for my condition. I found dialysis very painful, so I shifted to Nadiad. There was no change in my level of discomfort. My blood pressure had a tendency to rise suddenly and I would get cramps. All these issues were difficult to manage, but I was determined to continue my treatment.

Driving to Nadiad, feeling the needle prick, dozing away, waking up and driving straight to office was my routine. Life was busy. A discussion with my doctor led to a plan for a kidney transplant.

My mother willingly donated her kidney. Finance was arranged through friends and relatives and then, the big day arrived.

I recall how I was being wheeled away from my family into the operation theatre on 23rd November 2001. There was fear and some worry, but with complete faith in God and prayers, I went into the surgery. When I opened my eyes the next day, my transplant surgery had been done successfully. I had won my first battle. After 10 days in a special ward, I was discharged from the hospital.

Slowly, normalcy returned to my life. I worked hard to grow my business. But on 23rd March 2011, I was unwell and was diagnosed with a hernia. It was my second struggle for survival. I was operated upon for right inguinal with mesh hernioplasty, which resulted in swelling at the site of the surgery. Doctors waved it off as normal in some cases.

Three months after the surgery, I travelled to the UK with my wife and daughter. When we returned home, new health complications showed up. I got tired very quickly, suffered from chills and a slight fever. The feeling of uneasiness persisted all through that year.

In January 2012, I was admitted to the Nadiad Hospital because of an infection at the hernioplasty site. They did an aspiration and incision drainage to treat the infection. Samples of the drain's fluid were sent to check for tuberculosis and a Computerized Axial Tomography (CT scan) was done for fistula gram evaluation. The test revealed a colocutaneous fistula but there were no specific symptoms except some retention of pus. Other symptoms like stomach pain, vomiting and diarrhoea were not observed.

I needed regular dressings at the site for a year, so I drove to Nadiad every morning. Further investigation was done, leading to another operation to remove the mesh on 19th March 2012. Many other issues were still bothering me.

"How long will I live in 2 worlds, 1 in the hospital and 1 outside?" I asked my wife. She simply squeezed my shoulder, understanding my feeling, while her eyes expressed her own sorrow. Life was at a crossroads for my family!

Tests did not tell us much. Small operations and incisions were done. A blood culture of the pus showed Acid-Fast Bacillus (AFB) as positive. Following this, an Antituberculosis Therapy (ATT) was started to fight tuberculosis. This treatment continued for 9 months. On 18th February 2015, a fever with pain in the right hip region troubled my peace once again.

Another round of scans and Magnetic Resonance Imaging (MRI) were conducted. The culture showed the presence of gram-negative bacteria (Klebsiella) and kidney cancer (renal cell carcinoma) in the left native kidney. In June 2015, a nephrectomy was done and the left native kidney was removed. The wounds healed and I recovered. But the creatinine was rising gradually because of the medicine given for treating the bacteria, giving rise to another line of worry.

By December, I was experiencing severe pain and fever. I was hospitalised yet again. Another round of injections, reports, scans and operations began. I continued to experience some minor sensation pains, not much to report, but it kept me uncomfortable.

"How long should I remain strong? All these struggles are making me tired. I feel so frustrated! Since nothing is identified by tests, nothing is wrong, but I'm still in discomfort, with no solution found!" I thumped the table, silently relieving my grief.

My life seemed to be on 'pause mode.' A new pain bothered me, making it difficult to walk. I can't remember how many months I took Crocin thrice a day, without any relief. Then I was hospitalised for more than a month in Nadiad Hospital.

It was almost as if I had received a secret message; I decided out of the blue to go for a Computed Tomography (CT or CAT) scan on 9th May 2016. Suddenly, the doctors suspected that the intestine could be involved. I met a urologist. Another scan found a large abscess formation near the colon. A colonoscopy showed nothing untoward inside the intestine. The urologist contacted his friend, a colon rectal surgeon in Brooklyn, NY who suggested opening up to see if it can be operated upon and to understand what caused the problem.

In a major 12-hour surgery conducted on 25th June 2016, an abscess was removed and the colon was cleaned. The surgery was very risky but with all our prayers, it was successful. By God's grace, I sailed through it unscathed.

Though my recovery was handled well with the help of doctors, the creatinine stayed between 2.5 to 3mg/dl. Other reports were fairly average. I suffered from huge weight loss and lack of energy in those years.

After so many health issues, I'm left very confused about the unpredictable nature of this disease.

What amazes me is that a kidney failure in 1998 drove me through many dangerous rides, sometimes giving rise to hernia and tuberculosis, perforation of the intestine and even nephrectomy! It needed a doctor from the US to suggest opening up of the colon to understand the problem. In 5 years, my body passed through so many tests of life. Though it was a short span in my life, it was a medically intensive period, making it highly expensive too.

In my darkest phase, it was the light from God's powerhouse that made my struggle possible. In spite of agonising thoughts such as - *Will I be able to fight?* - people saw me smile and since they knew me well were confident that I would survive. Through many low phases, I was doubtful if I would rise above my problems. But today, I realise it was possible due to the dedicated family support coupled with my desire to live.

This is a thought that comes to my mind very often: *Battle is part of everyone's life. But a person who falls a 100 times, with the courage to rise again and never letting hope die, becomes a warrior!*

Nilesh B. Shah
Dialysis- 11 years
Transplant – 17 years

COMPROMISING A CAREER TO PROTECT A KIDNEY

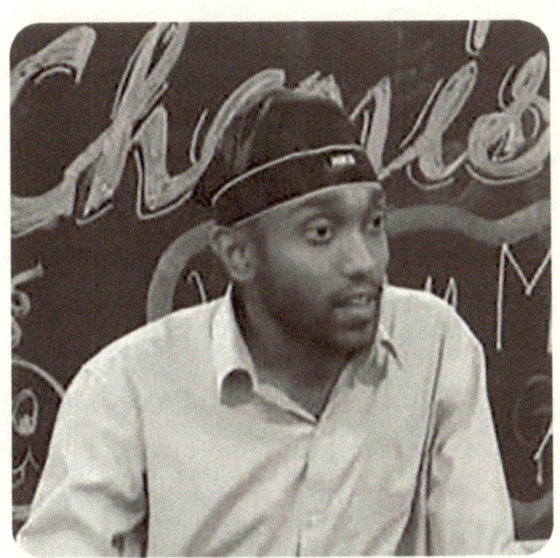

Hypertension

Many things happened to me in the past 2 years and it was all concerning my health.

My passion for organic chemistry led me to register for a post-doctoral study and I was in a 'happy mode.' To ruin this peace around me, my sinus had been playing up. The pain around my head and face persisted and finally, a visit to the doctor was scheduled. After an investigation, endoscopic surgery was strongly recommended to relieve me of the pain and help the nasal passage open up.

Just as I solved the sinus problem, I had a fall and a fracture. It just meant plenty of medicines and antibiotics. I was really annoyed and wanted my normal life back, with the research as my priority. But somehow, 'lady luck' had decided to desert me at this time of my life. Exactly what was going wrong came to be known only a year later.

It started with cramps all over my body. Very frustrated that I had to deal with another problem, I went to the hospital. The doctor advised a blood test, so I had it done, expecting to get some medication that would quell the cramps. With the report, I met the doctor. The doctor announced, "Your creatinine is very high. At 9mg/dl, you need immediate attention!" I looked at him thinking, *How did this happen?*

The doctor was talking and I suddenly caught the words, "Best treatment is a kidney transplant!" I looked at him incredulously! How can he talk about a transplant so very casually! I left his clinic with a smile and vaguely said I would discuss it with my parents.

My family was equally shocked upon hearing about kidney disease being my latest health problem. We took the reports and went to about 4 or 5 hospitals in Gujarat, meeting senior nephrologists there.

Everywhere we went, there was a similar response. My mother stepped in, offering her kidney without a second thought. So, we began the testing process, which included the blood group, cross-match and HLA typing. With all tests cleared and the donor's health being considered good to donate, the transplant became a reality.

At that time, a study protocol was being carried out for lesser immunosuppressants. I opted for this so that I would need minimum medication. As part of the clinical study, my dosage was less and the transplant was done at a concessional rate.

But complications chased me even after the transplant. I developed pneumonia. To cure the ailment, the dosage of some immunosuppressants was reduced leading to a tubular cell rejection. With great difficulty, the pneumonia was treated. My creatinine finally settled at 1.8 mg/dl.

I resumed my post-doctoral work with an aim to synthesise helically shaped molecules.

Though I was well for the next 1 year, it became clear that working with chemicals would negatively impact my health. One day, I was sitting at my desk. One cannot control one's thoughts, so mine strayed away. It was as if I was taking stock of all the unusual goings-on in my life. I never knew the exact reason for the kidney failure. No biopsy was done to find the cause. I wondered if the medicines for fracture and sinus had damaged the kidneys. I mulled over it for a long time.

Just then, my friend called and said, "Let's have tea. I need a break. It has been exhausting working right through the morning without any break!"

Over tea, he found me quiet.

"What's bothering you, Parvinder?" he asked.

I smiled with my lips, but my eyes were vague as I responded, "I'm at a stage which worries me a lot. I set out to work as a scientist with so much purpose and passion. But today, after a transplant, I'm no longer sure if I have chosen the right field."

"Working with chemicals such as hydrocarbons in their vapour state may create a negative impact on my transplanted kidney. You know most of the helical molecules and other chemicals, especially hydrocarbon solvents, are carcinogenic, which is not good for people like me whose immunity is suppressed by medications. What would happen to my health if I work with chemicals that are known to be health hazards?"

My friend listened and could understand the thought process. He nodded understandingly.

"When I was on dialysis, I thought I could not manage my research. I would get so exhausted and weak after dialysis, so I agreed to do a transplant. Now nothing is certain. I don't know if I should change to some other field which would not compromise my health."

"Parvinder, I can understand what you're trying to say. Looks like a complicated problem. But how will you solve it?"

"To me, sacrificing my dream is not something to worry about. Keeping my kidney healthy and alive is much more important. I can always find joy in any other field I choose. My priorities have changed."

I smiled back, now sure more than ever that my life was more important than a dream. After all, dreams are never real.

Parvinder Singh
Ahmedabad
Transplant - 3 years

LIVE LIFE IN FULL AFTER A TRANSPLANT

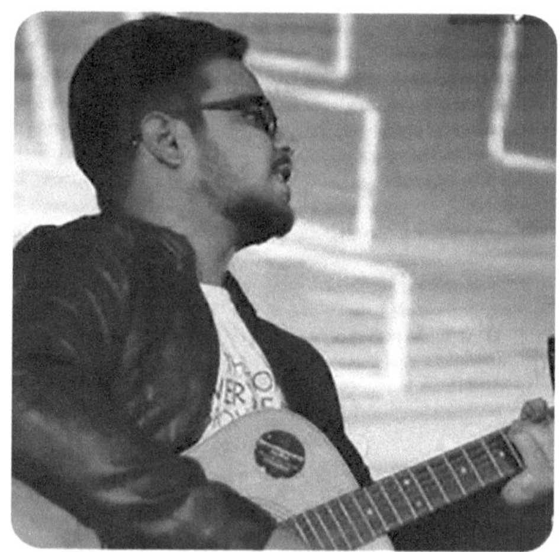

Hypertension

"The atmosphere in the hall was electrifying with music. It was amazing!" my brother said proudly. There, on the stage, I had sung my favourite song *Gulabi aankhein, jo teri dekhi*, with my fingers strumming the guitar. The flashing blue stage lights made it a perfect setting. As soon as I finished, there was a huge round of applause. It was an exhilarating experience – standing there and accepting the warm response.

Since my school days, I have been a performer. I did well in studies, got top grades, participated in all school activities and always inspired people around me to do better. But when I finished my class 10 exams, in spite of all my winning qualities, my mother was worried. "You must eat properly, you're not growing tall," she would nudge me, serving me another *paratha*.

"*Maa*, I'm not able to eat. I have no appetite. Sometimes I feel like vomiting!" I said this to stop her from serving more food on my plate. But when my loss of appetite persisted, she took me to a doctor, suspecting there was some problem with my stomach.

My mother made a decision; she would get a sonography done to check the abdomen area. My mother fixed an appointment and though I complained that I had many things to do, I went with her to clear all doubts.

Then we had a great shock! The technician mentioned that my kidneys had shrunk.

How we managed to leave the clinic, we can't remember. We took the fastest route out so we could breathe. Upon reaching home, all members of the family sat and discussed what was revealed by the sonography report. Together we decided our next course of action.

We were living in Rohtak, which is 70 km in the North West of Delhi. So, with my family, I went to Gurgaon to meet a renowned paediatric nephrologist. After several tests, the blood test result showed some unbelievable levels of important kidney indicators – creatinine was 14mg/dl and urea was 211 mg/dl. I was in a totally messed up condition. This news was not less than that of an earthquake for the family. We did not know what was happening.

My parents were very hurt. My father asked the doctor, "Sir, why do you think the levels went up so high? Our family only eats home-cooked food. So, I am unable to understand why Harshit is so ill. Why, at 17 years, is he facing kidney failure? This is a great mystery!"

The nephrologist explained, "This could be a condition from birth; it happens to many kids. They are born with such conditions. It is not due to something one has done or not done. Not due to any neglect."

My large family with uncles and aunts extended me their full support. They did everything to make me comfortable. It was decided that any 1 member of the family would donate a kidney to me. This gave me full confidence to face life. At no time was I left alone to wonder if I would survive. There was no chance for me to feel miserable. The family support was comprehensive.

In the next 1 month, the paperwork for organ donation was done. All the necessary tests were done and the day arrived very soon. My father donated his kidney.

I remember as soon as I was admitted to the hospital, many friends and family members came to cheer me up. It was as if I was going on stage for another performance. But I was only dressed in hospital clothes to enter the spotlight of the surgical ICU, where I would be centre stage of a life-saving surgery.

I was calm but was thinking, *I hope it goes off well. Very soon, I should go back to school.*

The surgery went well. The doctors and nurses explained to me how to take care of my health. They were all very kind. After surgery, I studied at home and prepared for my exams for 11th standard.

Today, I've finished my college education and work in Chandigarh, enjoying the comfort of family. My life's joys are restored and I lead a blissful life. I feel so blessed.

I performed in my college band. Music certainly makes me feel happy and keeps me healthy.

When life puts us in a hard spot, we must never ask God, "Why me?"

Instead, we must have faith, stay strong and say, "Try me!" Our being ready to face a challenge makes our life meaningful, as we will learn to lead from the front.

The phone rings and I say, "Oh, that's wonderful. When are we making the album?"

Now, I am planning my future. The kidney disease came into my life and I learnt a big lesson – to simply move on!

Harshit Bhatia
Haryana
Transplant - 5 years

NO SHORTCUT FOR SURVIVAL WITH CKD

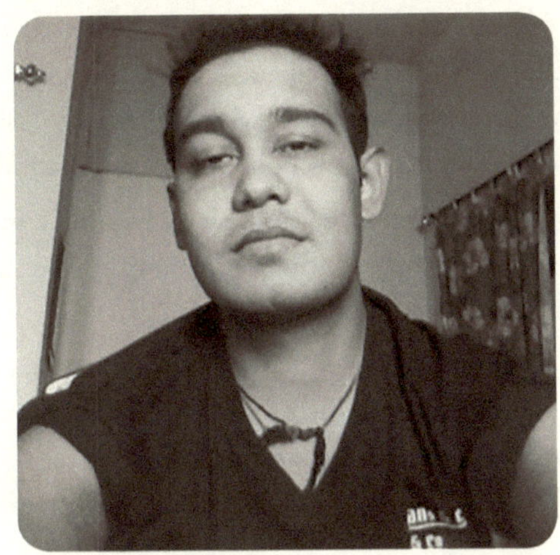

Hypertension

"What are you saying? Is it really possible?" my mother talked in Bangla. From the pitch of her voice, I could sense her excitement and wondered what my aunt was saying that made my mother so happy. But I was in a lousy mood as being on dialysis always left me grumpy.

"Yes, yes, I will tell Indranil and his father, and yes, we will come to Delhi soon."

Mummy came into my room, excited. "Indranil, Ishani auntie says she knows a doctor who can save the kidney, and it will be without dialysis! How wonderful *na*?"

"Is this true? Did *Masi* say so?" I said. My eyes were wide with disbelief and wonder but happy all the same.

"We have to meet him in Delhi!"

This was terrific news for us. So, we travelled to Delhi and met the doctor.

The doctor spoke with great conviction about how many people benefited from the treatment. We sat and listened to his talk, spellbound. Then suddenly, turning his attention to me, he said, "You can stop dialysis, my son. I know you must be facing so much pain." His words comforted me.

I could suddenly see an opportunity for an escape. Since the time I had fallen ill, I never had even a moment of joy.

My health problems started in 2004 when I was still in school. Like many other patients I spoke to in the hospital corridors, I had the same symptoms: loss of appetite and a feeling of nausea. I was also highly constipated. Within some months, I had noticed swelling in my legs. I was immediately rushed to the nearest hospital, and after a few tests, the doctor recommended that I meet a nephrologist.

After making several enquiries, my family decided to go to Christian Medical College, Vellore. After tests and a biopsy, the cause was detected to be membranoproliferative glomerulonephritis (MPGN). I was prescribed medicines and returned home to Dhanbad to take my school board examinations.

With great effort, managing the creatinine level with diet and medication for 4-5 years, I managed to postpone dialysis. But very soon my health deteriorated and as much as I wished otherwise, I could not escape dialysis.

I had heard of dialysis and how painful it was. I put up great resistance to starting dialysis. It was the toughest thing for me to accept. But my cousin convinced me that dialysis was important. So, I started the treatment with great hesitancy and was very unhappy with my treatment. To me, it seemed like it was the toughest period of my life.

But hearing the doctor advise me against dialysis, I was very relieved! He said it was a therapy and that meant no more dialysis!

Reality came to the fore only after 3 months of this therapy. A family friend brought to our notice that the doctor who gave me this mysterious treatment, which involved IV injection 3 times a day, was not a qualified doctor. About the time I received this shocking news, another problem surfaced. I had become seriously ill and had to be rushed to a Delhi hospital for emergency treatment! I was suffering from uraemia, with my haemoglobin down at 4.4mg/dl. It was indeed a miracle that I even survived.

After I became stable in 2010, I was fortunate to get a transplant. My father was my saviour.

But life with transplant had its fair share of problems. In 2016, I developed a lung infection that was diagnosed as tuberculosis (TB). In India, TB is said to be common among post-transplant patients whose immunity is suppressed with medications. To treat TB, strong antibiotics that were kidney-friendly were prescribed.

When I look back, I notice the many high and low points in my life. Wonderful doctors and hospitals saved my life at different times. But I can never forget the imposter who posed as a doctor. Getting some mysterious treatment nearly took my life.

For chronic kidney disease, following a single line of treatment is most advisable. There's no need to risk one's life by experimenting with treatments that your good-meaning friends or family members recommend. Always understand your treatment fully and then decide.

Today, for chronic kidney disease, only dialysis and transplant are recommended. They are seen as the best treatments all over the world and even in India.

Indranil

Dialysis: 4 months

Transplant: 8 years

UNEMPLOYED DUE TO KIDNEY DISEASE

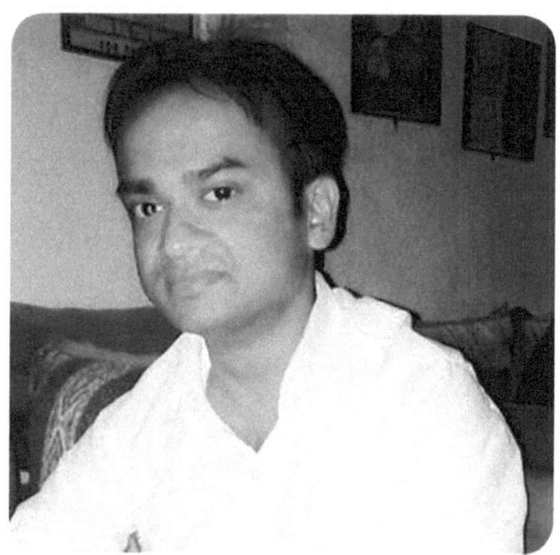

Hypertension

A tough period in life only gets tougher when one suddenly sees a familiar, stable environment disappear. I could almost see the big iron gates to my future close on me. It was a call from the Human Resources Department with the hard line, "Your continued absence from work breaks the employment rules. Your long absence from work is beyond the permitted leave period. I'm afraid we need to take some concrete action now."

I pleaded with them to give me some more time. At that time, it seemed important to do so. Today, I'm ashamed that I was begging with hard-hearted people when it was beyond their capacity to understand. "Please, can the company extend some special leave so I can recover? I really need help and support at this juncture."

The response was simply, "Extremely sorry, we can't extend."

Anger was my first reaction, but in some time, I began thinking of the circumstances that led to this treatment by my company. I also reflected on the past, which had lovely happy moments.

What happened to that carefree and happy life when I lived with my large family in Jharkhand in a household where being the youngest family member meant being showered with love? After schooling, I went to Pune to continue my education and completed my graduation there. I lived with my cousin in Pune, so I felt protected.

To specialise further, I registered for a master's degree in business administration in a renowned Pune institute. Later, I managed to get employment in a renowned MNC too. Life was almost how I wanted it to be: surrounded by a good supportive family and an exciting professional life. I had all the ingredients necessary for a good life!

Even before I was fully aware, changes happened in my personal life. It started with the graveyard shift from 2:30 AM to 11:20 AM. The odd working hours, with less sleep and changed meal times to stay awake, saw a gradual change in my eating patterns. I blamed my poor appetite on the inadequate sleep that disrupted my eating schedules. The office timing also resulted in less interaction with friends and family, so I was not communicating with people about normal things.

I had severe pain while urinating and passed blood, while headaches kept me irritated. Fear and lack of time made me self-medicate. How could I talk to anyone about blood in the urine? I felt lonely and finally, when it became unbearable, I shared it with my cousin who suggested that meeting a doctor should be my priority. I ignored it till my parents were called to attend to my poor health.

We went to a nearby hospital for a check-up. The doctor checked my blood pressure. Some tests were also done. It was shocking to see that the creatinine was double the normal range. A further check-up revealed I was at stage 3 of chronic kidney disease.

For a very long time, I felt confused, hurt and disappointed. Suddenly, my life was a mess. I was at crossroads, not knowing where to go or what to do. My family ran between cities, from Vellore to Ahmedabad, to understand how to handle the sudden detection of kidney failure. I was shown a rulebook that said only my parents, brother or sister could donate. My parents were both diabetic, and my sister had just become a mother.

My family almost collapsed under the shocking news, and they were heartbroken. Though we were confused, we began the search for a good doctor. Our next search would be for a willing and eligible donor.

I had resigned from my job to keep away from nagging office calls. Being out of a job meant all my dreams of a solid career were distant.

And then, a single beam of sunlight, a ray of hope appeared which made me feel loved again. A kind aunt came forward to give me her kidney. It is that precious moment of happiness that made me marvel at God. I was relieved.

While the testing process began, I also started dialysis. I was detected as Hepatitis C Virus (HCV +). It meant postponing the transplant till my blood was clear of HCV. Such setbacks put huge stress on a person waiting for a transplant. The suspense weighs heavily as one is not sure if one will get cured. Luckily, with some medical treatment, the HCV became negative.

Then, as soon as convenient, the doctor scheduled the surgery and my kind-hearted aunt donated her kidney. After the surgery, the enormity of the transplant made me grateful to God. I felt his blessings had made my survival possible. Gradually, all the fears I had experienced in the last year disappeared, my hopelessness began to recede and I developed positivity. There was renewed hope for life and a career. My family's bonding and the love showered by them made life worthwhile.

But in spite of precautions, I got urine infection after 5 months. With medicines, the infection was controlled but would return now and then. Creatinine was fluctuating between 1.3 m/dl to 3.75 mg/dl.

A biopsy of my transplanted kidney showed that HCV virus had affected it. My creatinine was stable, between 2-2.6mg/dl, but a doctor suggested that the virus could affect my liver.

But God came to my rescue once again. I got help from some Facebook friends. A reputed doctor in Delhi helped me with some good medications for HCV virus. The 6-month course of the antibiotics finally brought HCV under control.

To me, my career was always a top priority. I loved to be busy with work. When I got detected with CKD, I was handling a life-changing experience caused by the disease. It hurt me that I was forced to resign because I was unable to attend work.

After my transplant, when the new kidney created some health issues, I began to feel like I had lost all things that were precious to me: a chance to be employed and a working kidney. I felt very challenged. I felt very deprived.

Thank God now I have a working kidney and I work with a company. Life is fun again, but my lesson for life stays with me.

Manish Kumar

Author's note: For a person with chronic kidney disease, it is important to be in employment. It ensures that the treatments can be financed and the person's emotional well-being is maintained. Better understanding of the disease and some change in corporate employment rules will help.

IN SEARCH OF PARADISE

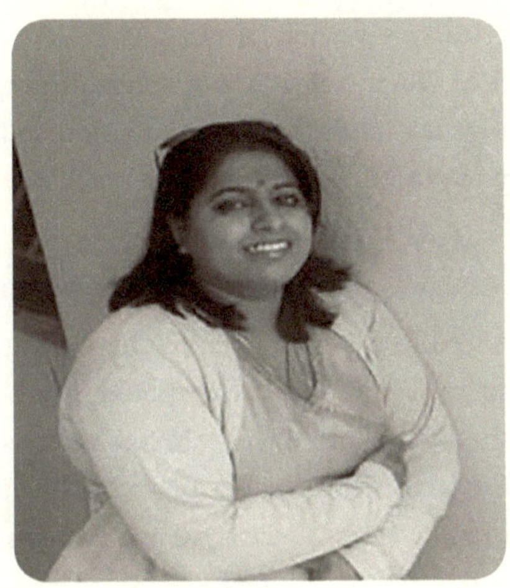

Drug Induced

I read about an interesting job offer from Unilever, with a posting in Florida. Yippee! I was completely ecstatic and was unable to control my joy. I quickly messaged my husband.

"Go, get it!" was his quick response.

I laughed and thought, *So amazing! How supportive can he be! He's letting me chase my childhood dream!*

By mid-afternoon, I finally sent the mail. After I sent my application, I could breathe.

I enjoyed my life and worked very hard to fulfil my dream. But a newly appointed manager wanted to implement her style of management, which also included recruiting new people to replace some of us. For fear of being terminated from service, I proactively began looking for a job. So, by responding to Unilever's vacancy, I was securing my future.

I had always dreamt of a career abroad, earning well and owning a house. For selecting a career option, I was keen on an engineering course but my family could not afford to pay the high fees, so I opted out. I certainly wouldn't like to selfishly burden my family. I reasoned with myself and settled down for a Bachelor's degree. It seemed my first dream was not compromised. It was within reach.

After graduation, fate sprinkled some magic dust on my career path. I began working for a call centre and moved into the IT Project Management department. There, I could see a great chance presenting itself to travel abroad for work. I was thrilled beyond limits. Then, the unthinkable happened.

My dad, who was diabetic, got hospitalised due to a medical emergency. We were all very worried. We needed to save him, so we put in all our efforts to work on his recovery. It was a period of worry, tension and constant prayers. I did some serious thinking. How could I leave my family in such a situation and leave India? I informed my office of my inability to travel. I owed my father full attention and support when his condition was serious.

It hurt me that I lost such a great opportunity. Maybe lady luck had deserted me.

I changed my job, moved to a company with a higher pay scale. On October 12th, 2011, while I was working late, my mother, who should have been asleep, staggered out of her room. She complained of breathlessness. Shockingly, as we entered the hospital corridors, she breathed her last. A healthy person dying like that was unbelievable. It was a cardiac arrest. Our family could sense the earth under our feet slipping away.

Back home, things changed too fast for me to grasp or react. My father had become very unsure of his health, so he found a suitable alliance and my wedding was fixed. Even as we tried to bring cheer into the family, another unfortunate incident happened to rock our boat. Within 2 months of my mother's death, my father took his exit, leaving us feeling orphaned.

My sister and I felt marooned. We were struggling to understand how to piece together our lives after the tragic end of our parents' lives, but surprisingly, we found some good people rallying around us. Maybe some magical dust was floating around. My fiancé proved to be a man with a great sense of humanity and a high sense of propriety. He stepped in and suggested we marry soon. With help from our extended family, my sister organised the wedding.

I enjoyed my new life with the wonderful man. In a month or so, I fell very ill. It was diagnosed as typhoid. Some very strong medications were administered to speed up my recovery. Thanks to my husband's good care, I was well. He kept encouraging me all through. I was simply overwhelmed.

For a year we enjoyed our life; it was sheer bliss.

On the job front, my application to Unilever was very promising. My gut feeling was that it would happen. But change is a norm of life. So, a few days after applying for Unilever, in March 2013, unexpectedly there was a swelling in my legs that made me very uncomfortable.

"Now what could this be?"

Assuming it to be a fracture, I went to an orthopaedic doctor. A painkiller was prescribed. By the next day, the swelling of my leg had become worse. I was advised a blood test. When my husband collected the report, the pathologist promptly alerted him, "Her creatinine level at 6.7mg/dl is very high. I think she should be immediately hospitalised as her kidneys have failed."

What he had said left us shocked beyond words.

I had never heard the word 'creatinine' before and the fact that I felt normal, with no symptoms of any kind, made me wonder why he had talked of something as dramatic as kidney failure. My career was now close to what I had dreamt all my life, so I rejected an unknown pathologist's opinion.

In a quieter moment, I decided to investigate my reports further. Second, third and many more doctors' opinions on the blood tests confirmed that I indeed had chronic kidney disease.

As soon as the last meeting confirmed it, Unilever's offer letter arrived with an amazing pay package for a 3-year contract, and I would have to stay in Florida.

The appointment letter ignited some great ideas as my ambitious streak re-surfaced. I spoke to my doctor earnestly, "Doctor, why don't we start the medicines? I have to go the US on an assignment. I'll follow the medication and take care." I used my brightest smile to make him decide favourably. I almost pleaded with him to toe the line with my unique plan.

The shocked doctor almost yelled, "You can forget your job; save your life first. You need to be in a hospital now!" He concluded, "If you want to be alive, you need dialysis."

At work, the manager felt justified when she talked sweetly about my health, but without any show of sensitivity, hinted that my work was suffering due to my health. Pursuing her line of thinking, she applied pressure on me to resign. She possibly didn't want a sick person around. I was not part of the organisational re-structure that was being planned by her. Repeating these discussions always put pressure, so when I wanted leave for a medical check-up it blew up into a big issue. With compromised health, the only option left for me was to resign.

In front of my eyes, the tall edifice of a life of comfort and reaching the topmost rung of the career ladder came crumbling down. For a very long time, I mourned the loss of such a wonderful opportunity. So, accepting chronic kidney disease became very tough.

Even as I woke up to reality, I realised that things had changed. My sister and relatives were maintaining a distance from me. It hurt me to have lost everybody while I was still coping with a conservative treatment. And miraculously, the people who held me together all through my health crisis were my husband and mother-in-law.

In some time, I began my Continuous Ambulatory Peritoneal Dialysis (CAPD).

In passing, the doctor mentioned that the kidney failure was drug-induced through the medicines I had taken for typhoid. It hurt me that my career prospects were destroyed. Even with minimum education, I had done well through hard work. With huge medical bills and no income, life was difficult. With great humility, I took a job with lower pay that gave me very little excitement.

The greatest blessing God granted me was to give me the most co-operative husband. He explained and made me understand why it was important to accept my disease. I am very grateful to God for giving me such a great life partner.

As an important step towards recovery, I registered for a cadaver transplant.

On 14th November 2016, I got my call. The call that brought all the hope back for a better life! Somehow, all my positivity was driven away by the uncertainty of waiting on the list for a transplant. But now, the hope has been rekindled. I don't know what the future beholds, whether I will be able to start a family and find lost opportunities or not. I am ambitious and want so much from life; will God grant me all that?

Kidney disease changed my life. It made me economically weak when money was most needed. Kidney disease does not mean the loss of mental capacity to perform, as the disease is more internal and physical, maybe at times. Many people on dialysis have managed their jobs and have been regular too. It is sad when educated people start judging a person's ability to perform a desk job without assessing all aspects and doing groundwork, like contacting the doctor for a fitness certificate. We need to be confident that management will show more concern and sensitivity. Such inhuman considerations bother me so much. In days when 'working from home' is gaining popularity, why is the world not seeing such alternatives for retaining sick people in their jobs!

I'm waiting for God's abundant blessings to put my life on track.

Nagamani Bharadwaj

PS: Sadly, Nagamani lost her battle. Post-transplant, she was hospitalised and succumbed to a serious infection.

A MOMENT OF ACCEPTANCE

Hypophosphatemic Rickets

I remember the time my mother, Uma, narrated incidents from my childhood. She spoke about it as their greatest moment of joy, "Appa and I were young, and you were our first born. Oh, how happy we were! The first moments were spent seeing you, marvelling at God's creation. Then we examined every part of you closely to see if everything was fine."

Unfortunately, not all deformities can be noticed by the naked eye, I suppose.

When we think of it, what can one say about parents' blind love? It always reflects the innocence of the babe nestling in their arms!

I was born to Uma and Suresh, a teacher and a scientist respectively. They rejoiced and planned small as well as big things for me. Life was wonderful, and they had no complaints.

As months passed and years unfolded, some uneasiness set in. Somehow, they felt my limbs needed more strength. My mother wondered at times if it had anything to do with my bones. Were they too weak? As I started growing, some signs of abnormalities came to my parents' notice.

Then one day, good news breezed into our home. My mother realised she was pregnant once more. The process of life, living and growing kept the family pre-occupied and immersed so that no early signs could break the mundane routine of our lives.

My sister was born. Now with a son and daughter, my parents felt their family was complete. I would spend time with my baby sister and chat away about many things that siblings like to share. I would touch her gently with my tiny fingers, scared of hurting her.

At some point, my mother could tell there was a difference between her baby Sita's limbs and my limbs but she shrugged the unpleasant thoughts away, believing it was her imagination. All was well until I complained of pain while walking.

This alerted my parents. Taking immediate action, my father fixed an appointment with an orthopaedic doctor who suspected a bone defect. Seeing the discomfort written on the adult faces, the doctor spoke of surgery.

Nodding, smiling and saying something incoherently, my parents left the clinic. My mother held me tight as if protecting me from surgery.

The couple faced some very uncertain times, not knowing what to wonder, what to do or say. They were worried more than before as now it involved the life of their firstborn. In my dark eyes, the pain was evident. But some wisdom prevailed, and they decided to wait for some time, instead of immediately taking the surgery route.

In a quiet moment, they consoled each other, "Maybe Paresh will outgrow it!"

The real comfort came from seeing my excellent performance in school. I was among the top 5 students in the class. I was full of wit and got into healthy discussions and would not lose ground in any argument. At home, my constant chatter with my sister and our special bond was always a delight to them. These small pleasures remained special moments of life, cherished and remembered.

At some stage, my physical health started growing into larger issues. My walk to school took great effort, and my classwork deteriorated, causing some concern to my parents. *Appa* took *Amma*'s hints seriously, and they headed to Mumbai's KEM hospital for a complete check-up. The doctor recommended some blood tests and a scan.

When the reports were received, my parents were stunned into silence. The blood test showed creatinine was 3 mg/dl, while the scan report shockingly revealed a single kidney instead of 2.

Amma was nervous. She could only say, "How can that be?"

Appa made her sit and said thoughtfully, "Never knew people were born with 1 kidney!"

The renowned nephrologist who attended to the case was a caring lady. She spoke reassuringly, "These things happen. Many people are born with a single kidney. Unfortunately, this single kidney is also affected by hypophosphatemic rickets, a disorder in which the bones become painfully soft and bend due to low levels of phosphate."

As the information settled in, my restless parents asked questions about all that was troubling them, "Now what will happen, doctor? What should we do?"

The kind doctor, being a very sensitive lady, was controlling her tears when she saw how my parents were so shocked and scared. Summoning some courage, she said, "Paresh's creatinine is 3 mg/dl. This means that his kidney function is decreasing. For the present, we will put him on medications, so that he is comfortable. Sometime later, we will have to plan the next stage of treatment."

Seeing tears threatening to flow from my mother's sad eyes, she added softly, "There's still time. You can take it easy, as it will take some time. Maybe even a few more years."

"I always felt my son found it difficult to go to school. I wish I had known this before," *Amma* whispered, her voice barely audible.

"Please see to it that he does not carry heavy bags… his bones are weak and it will be painful and may lead to further damage," the doctor said.

Next morning, while packing the bags and the lunch boxes, *Amma* suddenly cried. *Appa* tapped her on the shoulder and showed her the time on his watch. She hurriedly wiped away her tears.

Later that day, as *Amma* walked down the stairs with me, carrying the schoolbag, her suppressed emotions came to my notice. I tried diverting her attention with my chatter, but she barely heard what I said.

For an 8th class student, I had not grown much but I remained undaunted. My attitude won me many friends who willingly helped me. I would entertain them with tit-bits, trying to forget my pain when it was difficult to walk.

It was a gradual decline but suddenly, it escalated. One blood test showed creatinine as high as 9.4 mg/dl. The nephrologist, seeing my physical condition and low weight of 20 kgs, advised starting dialysis immediately.

Dialysis meant fixing a catheter. It proved to be a huge problem as my forearm's veins were far too thin. So, an access was created on my leg.

People would be sad seeing my parents take turns to carry me for dialysis. My weakness and frailty caused them so much anguish that my parents ignored all the attention directed towards us. Managing my health was their single purpose. This taught me to face my disease better.

Seeing me lying in a bed, tiny, with tubes connected to a machine, blood running outside the body and my big eyes filled with terror, left my mother overwhelmed.

"How can I watch my son in so much pain? Oh, he looks so scared!"

Releasing her anger, she said, "Let's do something. I can't watch this any longer. Look at the torture he faces during dialysis!"

The nephrologist's response was quick. "Kidney transplant is a solution," she said. My mother was determined. She said, "Yes, I will donate my kidney."

Without any delay, evaluation tests were conducted to see if there was a good cross and HLA match. In a few months, my mother donated her kidney to me.

I recovered under *Amma*'s loving care and my grandmother became a strong pillar of support throughout the period. The surgery attracted attention from a large number of family members, whose presence made a huge difference in our morale through the most challenging phase of our life.

I stayed at home for a whole year, settling in with the new kidney, observing strict hygiene and eating only freshly cooked meals.

When I resumed schooling, it was a long period of hard work. Eager to become self-dependent, I graduated in pharmacy. As a young man, I fought my way through crowded Mumbai trains, making sure to protect my kidney against any infection with a mask.

After I had worked so hard, suddenly it seemed as if I lost my momentum. Gradually, I became aware of the signs of the kidney slowing down. Blood tests confirmed my doubts.

When the kidney's function came to a sad end, I chose peritoneal dialysis. The new regime came with its own hygiene requirements. On peritoneal dialysis, there was a great threat of infections that could be very challenging. My family understood how the dialysis should be managed.

Amma, who had been a rock of support till now, felt the firm ground under her legs crumble. She felt the earth under her feet give way, and her anguish on seeing me back to square one became uncontrollable. As a mother, her pain was not due to my losing the kidney but because she was no longer able to run through a hospital corridor, fighting for my life. I could understand her mental trauma upon seeing me clamp the peritoneal catheter to the dialysate.

She was completely overcome by sorrow. The whole struggle since my childhood haunted her. She was inconsolable.

One day, she was walking while her mind was totally engrossed in the worry of how I would manage life while on dialysis. In an unfortunate accident, she fell down in the street. She was brought home and the doctor said, "She's jaundiced and her condition is serious. Give her good rest." But very soon she succumbed to it.

Seeing my life's strongest link break unceremoniously, I was deeply affected and fought hard to overcome my sorrow. *Appa* and sister eagerly helped me pick up the pieces of my shattered life and showed me how important it was to remain calm and strong.

Much later, I took on the role of a big brother and encouraged my sister, who was a promising dental student, to accept an internship. In the meantime, *Appa* began the search for my 2nd donor. Many friends and family members lent support and helped me. But the transplant was fraught with many issues. An acute rejection was treated with steroids and the graft survived for a short period.

By now, as an adult, with some imagination and innovative thinking, I arranged for my 3rd transplant.

Following the working from home (WFH) concept, armed with an MBA in finance, I entered the finance markets, picking up some interesting portfolios. My sister got married and settled down in the UK. Aware of my long-time interest in coins, she encouraged me to do research in numismatics. Later, she convinced me to apply for a fellowship.

It was a proud moment for my family when the Royal Numismatic Society, UK awarded me a Fellowship.

The close bonding between my sister and me made life very comforting for *Appa*, who missed *Amma's* presence dearly. He was aware of the important role she had played in building this wonderful camaraderie.

I am very eager about the projects I take up. Today, I travel between cities in South India to chase my dreams. Sometimes work takes me to Mumbai and sometimes I fly to the UK on some project. People treat me with great respect and regard as they judge me purely by my intellect; by what I can deliver and by my potential to live life on my terms, quite unconcerned about what anyone thinks.

I am now confident about meeting any challenge that presents itself. Life has become meaningful now, as I am closely working on kidney awareness programmes. Assisting a friend, I help in supplying low-cost medicines to patients in need of some support. Professionally, as a pharmacist, I work with a company supplying dialysis supplies to hospitals and clinics.

Memories of *Amma* building my fabric of life during my growing years will remain intact in my mind. *Appa's* rock-like support through every stage of my kidney issues is truly treasured.

Paresh

Dialysis: 2 months

1st Transplant: 9 years

Peritoneal Dialysis: 3 years

2nd Transplant: 7 years

Dialysis: 7 months

3rd Transplant: 8 years onwards

DIALYSIS, MY FRIEND

Nephrotic Syndrome

People on dialysis say that kidney disease ruined their life, career as well as marital status. I know it ruins everything. For me, it was actually like a friend who is with me for almost 15 years. I know it is hard for people who are new to dialysis, as it puts a full stop/pause to every aspiration in life.

Do not get disappointed, as there is nothing you can do about it. I too had breakdowns in my life but I never stopped my education. I completed my UG, with 4 hours of thrice weekly dialysis the past 15 years.

Try to always indulge yourself and in your interests to take your mind off dialysis. My interests are listening to music, playing games and reading, all of which help me when I am depressed. Now, dialysis has become a part of my life! Trust me, I had to go through a lot in my childhood. I too had a transplant in 2004, in which the kidney lasted only for 4 days. It had to be removed because it gave me severe cold.

Now, I just go to the clinic as though it is my 2nd home with patients and technicians who see me as a member of their family.

So, don't get depressed and believe in God. He always has a special plan for you. I would like to end with my favourite quote, as always, "NOTHING IS PERMANENT, NOT EVEN OUR PAIN."

BE HAPPY and take life as a GIFT!

Pramod Subramanyam
Dialysis: 10 years

DEFINING MOMENTS OF A TRANSPLANT

Glomerular Nephritis

The blood pressure monitor read 140/90. The doctor exclaimed, "It's very high!" When he suggested repeating the test the next day, it surprised me. I was a barely out of college, a shy, introverted 21-year old guy with a million dreams in my eyes, so it was a little confusing. It was an episode of nausea and fever that eventually brought about a diagnosis of a kidney failure. I was slated for a kidney transplant.

I vividly remember some incidents. I remember being wheeled into the operation theatre on 30th September 2008, within 8-odd months of being diagnosed with chronic glomerulonephritis. I recall that even in a state of trance, after the procedure, I gave a thumbs up to my dad. My mom had gifted me life a 2nd time. But beyond that, everything was a blur. I don't know exactly what I felt during that period.

A successful kidney transplant is like winning a small war in the grand scheme of things.

Life after a kidney transplant is different, to put it mildly, and is certainly not a cakewalk! It is important to realise and accept that all things will not go in our favour. But one must attempt to shape and mould the situations in our favour, to be in charge of one's destiny instead of being overwhelmed by circumstances.

After 9 years of my kidney anniversary, I can see many highs and lows in my life. I have seen periods of frustration and elation, optimism and pessimism, acceptance and rejection. Experiencing peaks of success and also crushing defeat, I could survive it all. I completed my chartered accountancy course even after 3 failed attempts. I pursued becoming a chartered management accountant and now plan to do a Master's in business management. I think my burning desire of fulfilling my teenage dreams is goading me on.

Each milestone achieved has taught me something. My quest for a life partner made me understand the biases general people had towards post-transplant persons. During such times, we must dig deep and trust ourselves without allowing self-pity and self-doubt to consume us. Finding a soul mate has helped me in being a better judge of people. My search gave me a wonderful friend and we are blessed with a lovely kid as well.

2017 has been a pivotal year in my life. I quit my overseas job when I decided to put happiness above every other objective and returned to India. I had over-stretched my energies, working long hours through weekends, which helped in understanding my physical and mental limitations. I also concluded that nothing is more important than family and health. As I write this soul-searching note, I quit again and am ready to embark on a journey of self-discovery in 2018. I don't know what the future holds, but it will be rewarding.

As human beings, we are all wired in a particular way. We always analyse our life with a "what if?" This is a futile exercise. Dwelling in the past, trying to understand why a particular situation happened or trying to chart out a path of life based on an arbitrary situation leads us nowhere. As in a game of cards, one has to play with the cards on your table and really believe in yourself. Only in that can one find happiness.

Sandip Singh
Transplant - 10 years

TRUE SECOND LIFE

Polycystic Kidney Disease

"Hi Dr. S, I'm told that both my kidneys need to be removed. Is it possible to do a single nephrectomy?"

"Of course, Sunanda. It can be done. Unless both your kidneys could endanger your health; generally, we start with the kidney that gives some problem," replied Dr. S, my kidney doctor. Little did I know then that this conversation would be the beginning of a life-altering experience for me, one that would make me view things, people, money, life and most of all the notion of God in a dramatically different way!

Somewhere there was a feeling of excitement in me, since after years of knowing that I was born with bad kidneys, after 2 years of dialysis with no visibility of a transplant, things were beginning to move. I had polycystic kidney disease, which leads to the formation of cysts that gradually destroy the kidney. The removal of one kidney would mean better health on the one hand and readiness for a transplant on the other. It was a step in the right direction and it gave me hope for a better life.

So, I decided to get proactive and planned the surgery. After checking out finances for the surgery, planning my work and leave schedule tickets to Mumbai for my brother and me were booked for May 13, 2015. Though I am not really superstitious, my mind started piling events and that could go wrong. 13th May was also Tuesday, believed to be unlucky and inauspicious. My brother Sanjeev and I were trying hard to break out of these beliefs and this trip was supposed to prove that effort. So, though these niggling thoughts stayed in my mind, I tried to block them out as best as I could. Was it some kind of premonition that was coming my way?

The hospital admitted me to a room on the 13th floor. Again, 13!

A dear friend came to see me as she was going out of town and was feeling very bad about not being there for me. Suddenly, her eyes welled up. I knew she was very perceptive and intuitive. "I am going to meet you when you return, so don't worry. Go on your vacation."

The next day was going to be a long day.

The surgery day started with doctor visits. My doctor came with anaesthetists, the chief cardiologist and his team of assistants, who collected my medical history.

The chief cardiologist informed me that my heart was not in a very good condition but a full cardiac would cover the surgery to take care of any emergency. I felt reassured with this detailed planning.

At around 12 noon, the ward staff arrived with a stretcher to take me to the operating theatre. "This is it," I thought. "It's all going to start now." The ride from the room to the OT reception area is the most confusing experience. You don't really know what to think as scenes from your life flash by. Your life somehow seems to be hanging in a limbo. I gave my brother a weak "Ta ta."

My brother responded with "Best of luck!" I thought I heard a quiver in his voice as we are just 2 of us looking out for each other. At the operation theatre the anaesthetists got to work immediately.

I saw impenetrable kind of darkness all around me. I was at a railway station and a train waiting at the platform. I ran towards a bogey that was crowded with people. I stretched out my hand and said, "Help me get on this train, I am unable to climb up." "No, no, go away! There is no place for you on this train." I fell down on the platform and the train moved away.

Then on a dark rainy night, I was on Marine Drive, standing drenched, feeling cold and miserable. Suddenly, I saw a taxi with a driver and the passenger seated next to him, who was my father. "Papa! Papa! Please let me get in, I am getting drenched!" I screamed. Papa rolled down the window and said, "No, no, there is no place for you here." I stood there feeling helpless, the rainwater and tears mixed leaving a salty taste in my mouth. The taxi drove off with Papa in it.

I could hear faint voices calling out to me, "Sunanda, you know, the good thing is that they are bringing you out slowly," someone said.

"Sanjeev, is the surgery over?" I asked my brother as I gained consciousness. My brother replied, "The surgery got over 2 weeks ago!"

"Two weeks back?" I said incredulously.

"Yes, a lot happened in those 2 weeks."

Dr. S stormed into the room with his team. "I am so happy to see you like this, Sunanda. We almost lost you. I am not letting you go again!" he boomed. The cardiologist walked in with his team, held my hand and said, "You have been through an ordeal, my dear, but you are a fighter."

I was bewildered. What was going on? Why were doctors saying these sorts of things? I asked for a cup of tea but I couldn't hold it. I had no strength. While my caregiver spoon-fed me my mind was questioning, "Why am I in this condition?"

I asked my brother what had happened. He was relieved, but sounded sad as he said, "In the ICU the doctors tried to find the cause for delayed revival. Your heart and lungs had crashed and you were put on an intra-aortic balloon pump to help your heart work and a ventilator to help you breathe. You had pneumonia with fever as high as 105 F. You were very, very critical and it was a touch and go scenario."

I was shocked. "How is it that I don't know any of this?" I asked.

"Because they had paralysed your body and kept you in deep sedation so that your heart and lungs could rest while the machines took over. They were doing dialysis for 8 hours – **Sustained low-efficiency dialysis** (SLED) and you were on round-the-clock life-saving antibiotics. You were being fed through a Ryles tube."

I couldn't believe this and wondered about the dark train and the taxi with Papa, who refused to take me on board. What was that? Why had I seen all that? Where had I seen all that?

In a flash, I realised that I had experienced near death, but it was simply not my time.

My brother had become very tense while I was in the ICU as doctors had shown little hope. While my brother silently wished and willed that I fight back, Dr. S literally ordered me to come out of it. I suppose all those wishes and prayers worked on my brain and my soul. Slowly, I began to recover.

I was on a road to a very slow, very painful recovery but I was alive. As I recovered I understood what we mean by the 'gift of life.' How wonderful being alive can be!

Today, I am thankful for the gift of a new life that I got from my doctors and my brother's determination to take me home alive.

Today, I feel the need to touch people's lives in whatever small way I can, to bring them some happiness and care.

Today, I have realised that money is very important in our lives, especially in emergencies.

Today, I do not fear death. When the time comes, I will go. There will be a place for me on that train or that taxi and there will be healing light all around me, not oppressive darkness.

Today, I know that love is the greatest force that heals and cures.

Today, I am truly living my cherished 2nd life!

Sunanda Brahma
Dialysis - 4 years

LONG FIGHT WITH COMPLICATIONS

Paediatric Nephropathy

17 years. Is it too young to have kidney disease?

Today, medicine and research show a growing population of kids and young adults affected by the disease. Paediatric Nephrology is rising, showing kids in the pre-natal stage are caught under the radar.

I began my journey with CKD at 17 years of age. My father too had suffered and he succumbed to the disease. In my case, the doctors claimed it was a hereditary disease.

I was with stage 3 nephritis. Instead of buckling down, I decided to fight the disease, so I joined the Bangalore Engineering College, for computer science, even when I was strapped to the hospital bed for 3 days each week for dialysis.

With great determination, I not only qualified but also became the topper. I was selected during a campus interview and was much sought after by many top companies. My compromised health was a reason for worry but they appreciated me for my intellect and my ability to process high-level data. I was involved in the development of cloud computing for my company, giving them an edge in the market.

I was always busy with clients from Europe and the US on outdoor meetings, attending as many as 5 meetings a day!

One day, I met a middle-aged lady at the dialysis centre. After meeting me on several occasions, when we had exchanged many interesting conversations, she said earnestly, "What makes you stand out? Is it what you speak? Is it your intelligence? Is it your courage?

"You, my friend, are not a conversationalist, yet you are a great winner. You fought your disease as best as you could. There was a failed transplant. Thereafter, you spent 15 years on dialysis, which meant some complications. You contracted HCV, anaemia and thyroid induced tachycardia, fluid and acid retained. What makes you, my friend, stand out?

Your charities extend to partial funding of 3 regular schools, 1 blind school and supporting 15 patients for EPO injections and dialysis. People like you need to be celebrated."

I was glad to get her handsome tribute.

SR

****

This is a story based on real incidents in a dialysis patient's life. As of 6th October 2015, his cell phone buzzed but he had stopped talking to me. The fluid collected in his abdomen was sent to a university in the US for testing. Under the scanner, the fluid showed millions of bacteria. His abdomen was swollen, almost like advanced pregnancy. It was tough to carry so much fluid and walk. Removing the fluid was a painful experience, but he would see it fill back in the abdomen. This condition began in October 2014 and he has been facing his end-stage for almost 6 months.

He visited the group some months back to speak with his friends. Now, he wants to be left by himself. God bless him.

RAN MY LIFE'S RACE

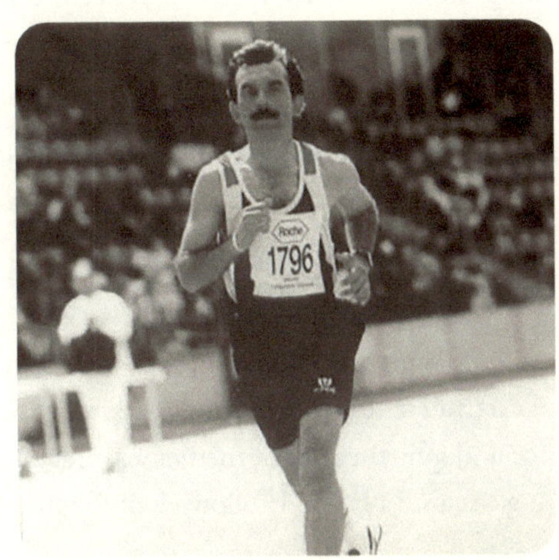

Hypertension

"When, at 36 years, I accidentally found out my kidneys had failed, of course, I was shocked! It took time to understand and implement my plan for survival," he said simply. Many of his friends gathered around him knew that his words were full of conviction and he made a statement of purpose. This was at the Bundh Garden, where the group met once a month to share their progress post-kidney transplant.

One man approached him and asked, "Vasu brother, tell me a little more. How did your family react?"

"Worried and shocked! But very soon, my mother offered her kidney. The next thing is all my brothers and sisters wanted to donate."

"You're lucky, brother. Who was your donor, Vasu?"

"My nephrologist found my mother as the most-suited donor. In a few months, I had a transplant. What about you? Who was your donor?"

After letting out a sigh, he said, "Vasu brother, at first no one offered me a kidney. I was on dialysis and when my condition deteriorated, my brother donated."

I realised with some pride that I was indeed lucky. "I too had dialysis for some time. It was bad but ultimately, it was all fine. I'm sorry, brother, for your delay in getting a transplant. But this is the case for many people here." I pointed to people in the meeting and said, "It's the same story. What to do? People are scared to donate. So, one has to be happy when someone finally donates to keep us alive." I patted his shoulder and started moving around.

Someone was talking about diet, so I stood there, listening. He was talking sensibly, saying moderation and hygienic home-cooked food were best.

In another corner of the garden, someone was upset. So, I walked over.

"You know, it's tough to manage maintaining a transplant. My friend lost his transplanted kidney yesterday!"

As soon as I reached there, someone asked me, "Vasu brother, how have you maintained it for so long?"

I smiled and recalling some incidents, mentioned calmly, "Soon after my transplant, many people narrated stories of kidney failures. So, I decided to strictly follow my doctors' advice and guidance about medicines, diet and water consumption. Within a year, everything became a habit. I followed all the do's and don'ts."

Just then, someone called out to me.

So, I said, "Instead of worrying, if we become disciplined, everything will be alright."

Excusing myself, I went to the other group. I joined the discussions there and then went to sit on a bench by myself.

I thought of my life. Born in a simple family and educated in Ballari, Karnataka, I was working in a private company when I was diagnosed with ESRD. The kidney transplant happened on 11th March 1992. Thereafter, I never paused to wonder about the lightning that had struck me. That's how I reached my 26th-year post-transplant. Some credit for my kidney's maintenance rightfully goes to my wife, Padmavathamma, and to my wonderful children. They added so much happiness to my life that I never ever felt sad about going through kidney failure.

Kidney disease changed my life, but I took it in my stride and moved on to do some good work for the society. I made friends with people connected with kidney diseases. I got introduced to the founders of Kidney Patients Welfare Association (KPWA). Seven transplant recipients formed this Trust on 13th September 1991. Eager to help people who were unable to manage the disease due to economic considerations,

I joined the organisation and became very active in advancing the group's work. About 525 members got registered with the KPWA from the southern states of India.

Among the new friends I made in the process, I had a friend from Novartis, who supplied Cyclosporin – the immunosuppressant that was prescribed to all post-transplant patients. He casually talked about the World Transplant Games (Olympics for Organ Recipients). This got me interested. I was basically a sportsman who had played a lot of cricket and participated in athletic events during my school years.

Keen to participate in the next transplant games scheduled in Manchester, England, in August 1995, I started practising. The small hurdle was, I didn't possess the organiser's address, though I was aware they were from Manchester.

Without any hesitation, I wrote a letter to 'The Organiser, World Transplant Games, Manchester, England' requesting them to send the details and procedure of participating in the games. By a stroke of luck, I got a reply from Dr. Mourice Slapak, the president of the World Transplant Games! The details for registration came but luck seemed to be short-lived. The deadline for submission was too close to complete the formalities required to participate, like organising funds and travel visa. With a heavy heart, I missed this golden opportunity to represent India.

Meanwhile, my doctor, Dr. Siddaraj, connected me with Dr. R.V.S. Yadav from New Delhi, who was organising the All India Transplant Games in September 1996 in New Delhi. Serious practice began, and with a small team of 13 transplant recipients from KPWA, we attended the game. In a twist of fate, all my team members won medals, except me. While trying to avoid a participant who fell across on my track, I broke my right ankle.

Kidney disease taught me not to give up easily. I wanted to participate in the next World Transplant Games to be held in Sydney, Australia, in 1997.

With guidance from Dr. Sankaran Sundar, I contacted a medal winner in Asian games, Mr. Sunil Abraham and Mr. V.R. Beedu, a well-known coach. They agreed to coach me. Under their special care, I trained to compete with other regular sportsmen who were seasoned participants.

I received training for 100 m and 400 m, with long jump as an additional event. Finding a sponsor became the next hurdle. But with some effort and friends' help, I got connected to Mr. Syed Kirmani, the national cricketer, who helped me in getting sponsorship from the State Bank of India.

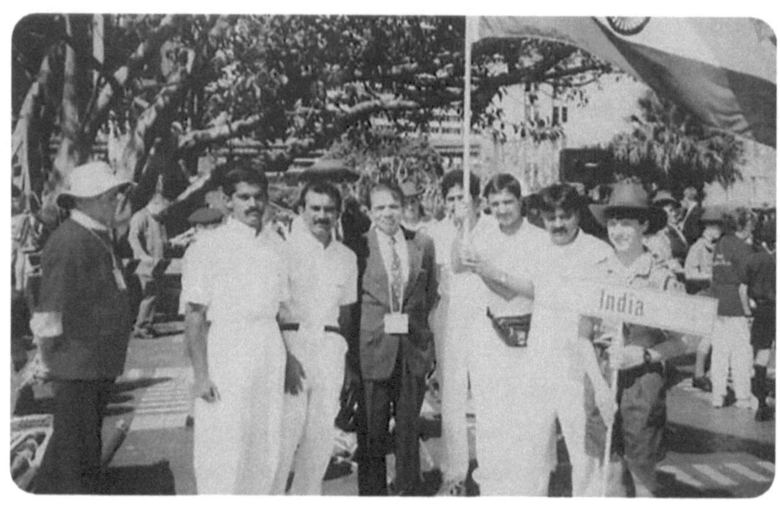

A 5-member contingent, along with Dr. R.V.S. Yadav and Dr. P.K. Sarin travelled to Sydney in 1997 to participate in the XI World Transplant Games.

I lost in the 1st heat/round participation in 100 m and long jump, but I felt consoled that my performance was the best among other Indian players.

Then I managed to reach the finals of 400 m. After 3 heats and a semi-final, I won the 6th place with a record of 68 seconds. I was the only Asian to reach the finals in that event. I participated in 1500 m race but was the last to finish.

In September 1998, Dr. P.K. Sarin organised the 1st SAARC Games in Amritsar. Participants were from Sri Lanka, Nepal, Bangladesh and Bhutan. I finally got the top positions! I stood 1st place in 400 m and 2nd place in 100 m.

We began facing financial constraints, and the lack of sponsors meant that only Mr. Nidhi Kanth Jha, from Patna, and I could participate in the XII World Transplant Games, held in September 1999 in Budapest, Hungary.

I managed to reach the quarter-finals in 100 m, finals in 400 m and in sprint, I got the 5th position.

In the next games at Kobe, Japan, I was offered free participation by the organisers, but I fell sick with septicaemia, so I could not participate.

For the next games to be held in France and Canada, Mr. Bala Kumar, from Coimbatore, and I were ready, but we were denied visas for both the games. I took up the matter very seriously with the World Transplant Games Organising Committee; the visas of the participants should be arranged by the embassy of the host country.

I could not participate thereafter due to financial issues.

In the Trust, KPWA too I am challenged for raising funds. Many members require financial assistance and we are unable to assist them on time. We approached the Government for help, but to no avail. Through a newspaper, I made an appeal to the public for contributions.

The road is long; each day is a new beginning. I keep running to my next goal – to see more patients survive.

Vasu Sandur
Transplant - 26 years
Managing Trustee of Kidney Patient Welfare Association
Executive Committee Member, Kidney Warriors Foundation

TRANSPLANT, THE REALITY

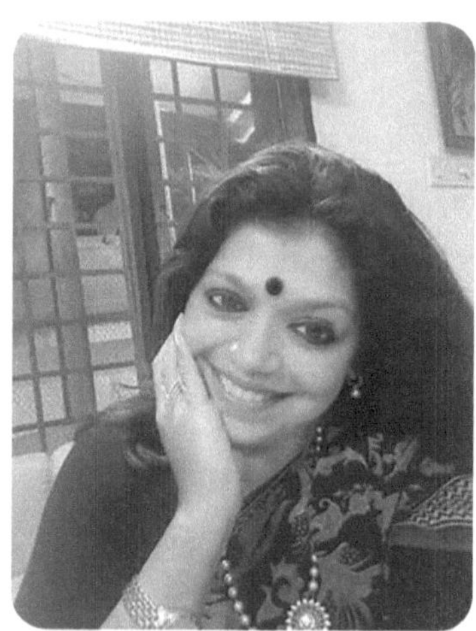

IgA Nephropathy

Life is full of ups and downs, and as David Michie says in his book *The Dalai Lama's Cat*, "It is not so much the circumstances of our lives that make us happy or unhappy but the way we see them."

It does sound easy to write and read but I'm sure in the back of your mind, you will never think that life will make you face anything out of the ordinary. So, we don't know the plethora of emotions that would arise in a given life-threatening circumstance. But as you turn a different corner, your life could actually change so permanently that your past will seem to be a dim memory.

The only thing we knew as a family about organ donation was that 26 years ago, my *mamama* (grandmother) had donated her eyes. We knew nothing more and somewhere deep in our hearts, her act always kept us inspired. You never really think of needing an organ donor. Maybe sometimes it can cross your mind to donate an organ like my grandmother did.

You never meet people by accident. They always come into your life for a very definite purpose. The purpose is only revealed later. That's exactly where my story begins. And it was a startling revelation.

On a regular day at an organ donation awareness meet, I ran into Dr. Philip. G. Thomas, who was heading the transplant unit at the time. We kept in touch and over time, I realised that he had written a book called *Transplant Story*, a book about the miracle of life and how the donor is really the true hero in a transplant case.

After reading the book, I told him that I was deeply moved by the book and was ready to do anything to help organ donation. Little did I know that the very next day, my brother was going to be diagnosed with IgA nephropathy and that 90% of both his kidneys had stopped working! Incredulous as it may sound, that's exactly how it happened. Our world was spinning without a stop. My family didn't know what had hit them, as it does for most families.

My brother had to be admitted to the hospital and a battery of tests was performed on him. The 1st set of tests determined that my brother needed dialysis. For that, he needed a fistula. But the fistula fitted on his left arm didn't work, so there was a temporary catheter in his neck. This then got converted into a permanent one.

The next step was a set of biopsies that revealed that transplant was the only step forward. Reading a book and getting inspired to help is one thing but when that story becomes your reality, it takes life to a totally different level. *Transplant Story*, of course, deals with a liver transplant through a cadaver donor, but the process, the pain and the poignancy are still the same.

Learning about CKD

Countless hours of sitting outside the dialysis room makes you gravitate towards fellow 'bystanders'; the term used for people like us who wait for their loved ones outside. ('Caregivers' would be a better word and more appropriate, though.) Guided by the *Transplant Story*, while sitting, I chatted with fellow bystanders and this actually helped me understand a lot more about my brother's condition.

My conversations with Mary Teacher, Maya, Usha and Leena all revolved around the effects of urea, potassium, creatinine and sodium on a dialysis patient. Each kidney patient had some sort of a kidney failure but the causes were different. Our conversations ranged from IgA nephropathy to Ayurveda, from diabetes to hypertension and an amalgamation of medical jargon, which at that time was far too difficult to comprehend. But, as caregivers, we were united by common concerns and experiences, so there was a desire to know more.

Conversations moved onto exchanging notes on how to leach vegetables. How much water is the right amount? Is itching due to a phosphorous build-up? Or was it just a side effect of dialysis? What is heparin and how many litres of filtration happened? Was the dialyser changed every time? Was sleep a problem? And anger a side effect? Oh God, the list was endless and exhausting.

But all these discussions gave us answers perhaps no book or medical journal could have given us. The reason being, it was the advice and information from likeminded people who had only a single purpose in life and that was to enhance the quality of life of the family member who was ill. Most bystanders didn't like asking questions but warriors like Leena, Maya, Tom's father and I always had questions. We got lucky; our doctors were concerned and always ready to support our growing curiosity and of course, telling us when we were fumbling. Countless coffee sessions with doctors and the numerous support groups on the Internet also helped me greatly. Facebook faces a lot of flak, but it was actually quite a turning point as the communities involved in transplants were always there to share and discuss issues.

It is well-known that a patient cannot go through all this by himself or herself. They need a 'champion' of sorts to help them face the trauma of a near-death experience, especially one who is in the end-stage of the disease, needing a transplant. But these so-called 'champions' also need support and truly, the number of people who step in does add up to a personal little 'village.'

Once we had a transplant scheduled, it was important to understand the post-transplant issues. I became aware of the implications of being on immuno-suppressants, this meant that my body's immunity was compromised; steroids and their role; to watch for levels of Tacrolimus (TAC) in blood; relevance ultrasound scans and constant monitoring meant life-long responsibilities.

Taking the Lead

My brother was not married. My parents did have a home here in Kerala, though we were settled in Calcutta. A very secure safety net had to be woven to get our family to embrace the trials and eventualities of transplant. I took it upon myself to be the 'contact person' for everything. From being in the hospital on alternate days for dialysis to managing the home on the other days, while my husband just took over the responsibility of the children and home, I was able to manage it well.

To my surprise, my daughter totally busted the myth that a mother being at home was directly proportionate to good results in the class 10 exams. My daughter managed her entire 10th with me not being there and made us proud by coming out on top with a perfect 10!

My parents were able to deal with my brother's brush with CKD better because the faces of their grandchildren kind of cushioned and took the sting off the horrible reality they were facing.

My Brother and His Health

The days at home meant friends and relatives pouring in to see my brother. A decision was taken to make the home environment a happy place because apparently smiling in the time of adversity 'boosts your immunity.' So, it was a happy home and my brother was slowly getting stronger with exercise, love and a controlled diet, to run 'the biggest marathon of his life.'

As my brother lay in the dialysis room or post-surgery in isolation, he would have dealt with his own demons. There was really no way of knowing what was lurking in his mind but I decided to keep asking.

The day of the surgery was fixed as the 15th of October. Slowly, things fell into place. I recall the time we faced a new challenge of finding a donor. I could be one as my blood group matched. But if not me, for any reason, who and how? These times felt like a roller coaster ride that you remember getting on to, but when you got off, you were unable to fathom ground reality.

The process to register on the cadaver lists in the hospital and on the Kerala network of organ sharing (KNOS) was another aspect to be handled. As I dealt with it, there was more to learn about blood tests, antibodies, plasmapheresis, altruistic donors – related/unrelated/cadaver donor, so I bounced questions all around. A 'negative result' added to our grief. Then, what a relief! I learnt that in medicine, all reports having 'negative' is a good sign, except in the case of pregnancy!

My brother's IgA nephropathy was an aggressive one, so till it became dormant through active dialysis, he was unable to go for a transplant. If he were to receive a cadaver kidney, frozen biopsies would tell us whether the retrieved organ would be suitable.

Live donor meant blood tests, full body check-ups and scans of the kidney. These lab results would rule out antibodies, disease and tell us the size of the kidney, its filtration rate and how many arteries were involved. If I thought this was an alien language, the paperwork was going to shock us into oblivion.

All medical and personal details of the donor and recipient were in a file to be submitted for police verification, panchayat approval and a no-objection certificate from the family. Then the task of facing 2 committees! One at the hospital and one at the district level to make sure everything was in order and legal. Being in Kerala was a blessing because people and systems here are more proactive and we were dealing with an educated population.

The transplant finally happened. My brother found an altruistic live, unrelated donor.

Rooms at home had to be sanitised and learning to say 'no' became my new mantra in order to maintain hygiene and a safe atmosphere. After the transplant, he had to take medicines every day at the right time. The donor, who also risked his life, was up and about in 3 days. We made him stay for an extra 3 days so that he could become stronger and be in better control. That also assured his wife that he was truly very important to us. The donor had to deal with not working for 3 months, but for my brother, the saga continued for 10 months. The feeling of not being valuable and in control played heavily on his mind. However, the love and happiness slowly cleared out quite a bit of those insecurities. Now, he's busy playing golf as I type, sitting on the lush greens of the Royal Calcutta Golf Club during the enchanting Kolkata winter.

Cadaver Transplants Are Crucial

During the process of acquiring details, I realised how important it was to have a donor. Cadaver donors (deceased) are truly a blessing. However, many stigmas are attached to it by the society in the name of religion. For me, however, if you can give your body parts after your time, there is no better *karma*. Then, of course, there is an argument about brain dead people and how they are being perceived. Many people believe their loved ones are declared brain dead so that the hospital can add one more successful cadaver case to their list. But this is not true. The hospitals follow the rules for declaring a person brain dead. Doctors work round the clock to look after such cases. Many departments from Critical Care to Neurology, along with surgeons and nephrologists, work together to do the right thing.

The transplant coordinator is yet another unsung hero, who actually goes out there to help and explain to the recently bereaved family about how their family member could save so many lives. Emotions run high during such dialogues. Questions keep cropping up. There's always a lingering doubt of the person coming out of being brain dead and also if the person wanted to donate. Therefore, during our lifetime, if we pledge to become organ donors and our families are made aware of the decision, I feel the trauma would be less.

It will be interesting to know that a cadaver donor makes it possible for transplantations of organs such as heart and pancreas, and combinations of organs (like simultaneous kidney-pancreas or simultaneous kidney-liver). For these organs, live donors have no role to play.

Thinking about 100s of people dying because they haven't been transplanted at the right time becomes the basic reasoning for signing up for organ donation. There are truly so many lives to be saved.

Financials

To add to all the issues around the disease, this is one side no one realises till the bills start hitting you. We were lucky that my brother's company had given him total insurance but still it was, at times, crippling and catastrophic. Day-to-day expenses! Logistics of travel! Follow-ups with doctors and check-ups! All of these added up. It occurred to me that many people are not adequately provided for to meet the financial challenges.

Finding My Peaceful Moments

There were times when I actually went on my knees and said, "Thank you once again, God, as it could have been worse." When finding a donor was a challenge, I truly believed, once again, in the power of prayer and God Almighty. And truly, what doesn't kill you only makes you stronger.

It was not easy but definitely becomes easier when you don't think about illness as a punishment for your sins. Being thankful and being well informed, with a great set of doctors to rely upon made the whole process manageable.

Smiling at the guards and engaging in conversation with the canteen staff, cleaner, dialysis unit technicians and even the barber, Mohanan *cheta*, gave us many insights and lots of the hope. Our village population rallied around, so we never lacked support.

Our tryst with destiny and the transplant world through my brother's kidney transplant motivated me more to be an organ donor. Though I had already made up my mind to donate my organs after reading *Transplant Story*, my daughter Ayesha's school campaign on organ donation was yet another reason to strengthen the purpose.

Sitting in the hospital for months, I got to see first-hand how a bereaved family put away their sadness and embraced happiness and joy when they realised their deceased family member, through death, had given life. That emotion I saw is something one probably experiences during childbirth. Will it work out right? Will it work out wrong? All such questions recede into the background because life is precious and worth a fight.

For me, my brother's altruistic live donor, Subhas *cheta* (older brother in Malayalam), and many such donors, including the cadaver donors, are real heroes. In my eyes, they are close to God, as are the doctors who make sure everyone gets their share of life. It's not necessary for all of us to burn our fingers to know fire. But learning from others who saved a life through a transplant should be reason enough for all of us to become organ donors.

"Science has no substitute for courage" and to that I add, "Courage can change the face of science... so become an organ donor."

Anjali Uthup Kurian
Dialysis: some dialysis
Transplant: 10 months
Dialysis: ongoing

INSPIRED TO WORK FOR KIDNEY PATIENTS

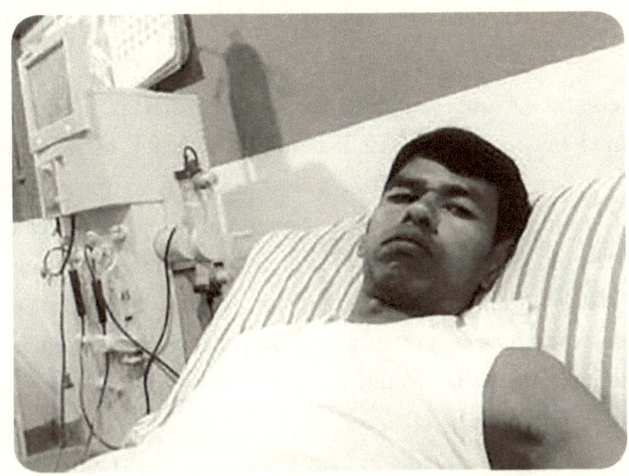

Hypertension

Who can ever say, "I expected my kidneys to fail"?

I wonder! As for me, I least expected that my life would change in the next few days after the diagnosis. It started in 2012. I had lost my kidney functions completely and needed to start dialysis soon. I had no time to assimilate, think, wonder and plan. So, slowly, as I was moving around getting tests done, I was getting ready mentally to be connected to a machine to purify my blood. The initial shock of the disease led to lots of physical and mental adjustments, leading to many financial implications.

I was working with the Taj Hotels & Resorts Group as a spa therapist. It was a job that simply matched my personality. I enjoyed the job; people loved and respected me and the money was coming in. Life was wonderful and I would often ask myself, "What next in life?"

But overnight, everything came tumbling down. Such happiness was in the distant past, some sort of a dreamlife that will go down in my history. Kidney failure brought about many changes in my life. My attitude towards life changed seeing the harsh realities of life; the truth is that one loses so much of one's life in a single stroke. Times with friends changed, as now friends were people struggling with a kidney disease. My physical condition had changed. And yes, financial status too!

With dialysis, I was busy pursuing small freelance jobs for money. Gradually, through the time spent alone on the hospital bed, my mind kept churning out thoughts, ideas and aspirations. Apart from thinking of earning revenues, it went into what was needed to be done to raise awareness about the disease. Two big things for people wanting a transplant are a donor and finances. Both are needed! Many have one and not the other. As an individual who has neither, how would the person find the road to happiness?

Above all else, great family support through the disease, especially with a good diet and sustained healthcare is crucial! I quietly watched as many dialysis friends were deserted by family members because there was no material gain from the patient. Instead, money was spent for the person's upkeep. Some of them didn't get nutritious food to compensate the loss of protein and nutrients during dialysis. Good food is needed for maintaining health condition. Being deprived of protein and low in haemoglobin meant they were constantly on protein supplements, iron injections and erythropoietin (EPO) that would further increase medical expenses or lead to increased chance of complications.

Then I decided to look around at positive things happening around me. I noticed that in Kerala problems were fairly simple. Lots of things were happening around kidney diseases. Live donor transplants were quite easily accepted. The country was seeing changes. **Green corridors** were used to reach organs fast. Cadaver transplants were happening. I dream of a day when people become willing to donate a kidney as they donate blood. It is a change that will happen gradually, but we must create the awareness.

With such a determination, I decided to work for the community to bring changes in the lives of kidney patients.

The opportunity to work with kidney patients soon opened up when I met some chronic kidney patients who, like me, were undergoing dialysis and were planning to form an association. I got actively involved with the activities of this patient support group; we even organised World Kidney Day, free health check-up camps and organ donation awareness campaigns.

Life is beyond dialysis. It's about spreading information. I have never turned back.

But with intermittent health issues that happen during dialysis, my constant prayer is to stay strong.

Jerry Rodrigues
Dialysis: 5 years

DIET AND EXERCISE ARE IMPORTANT FOR LONG KIDNEY LIFE

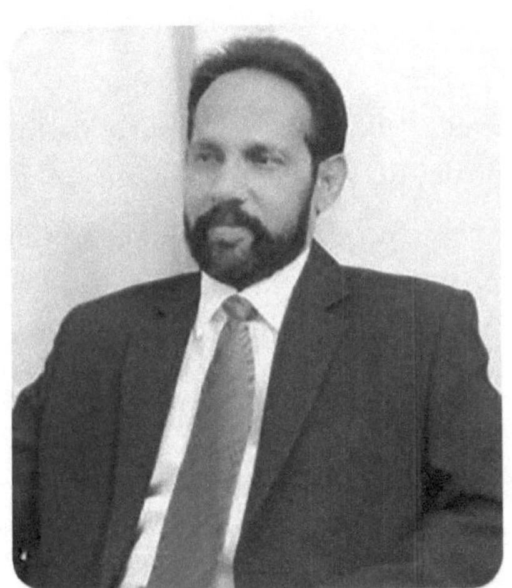

Hypertension

I was travelling by train from Madurai to Guruvayur. Pangs of hunger were driving me insane. Our train was running late, and we were in Nagercoil station for about an hour. Vendors were around selling food packets. I saw my co-passenger open his meal as I returned to my reading. He nudged me and said, "Brother, why don't you share this sandwich with me?" I thanked him and requested him to go ahead and eat.

But it did not stop there. After washing down his meal with a cup of tea, he continued his conversation, "Everyone is eating on the train. Are you observing a religious fast?" Normally, I would not entertain such conversations, but I saw compassion in his eyes. So, I began talking, with some passion, and I could see his eyes widen in surprise.

"I have had a kidney transplant and need to eat freshly cooked food."

"What?"

Then over the next 1 hour, my whole kidney story was disclosed.

"It began with a serious road accident in 1987. But a year later, some symptoms surfaced.

Though I was rushed promptly to the hospital, the doctors couldn't identify the problem. After seeing many doctors in Kerala, in desperation, I went to 1 of the most reputed hospitals in Chennai. They did some tests and quickly found the problem."

"What did the doctors say was the problem?" he asked quietly.

"It was a kidney failure," I replied softly, seeing him concerned.

"This must have been shocking!"

"Yes, brother, my family was shocked. They never expected this."

After a pause to recover my composure, I continued, "The doctor started me on dialysis as further delay would endanger my life. My mother and wife were praying and observing fasts and finally, my mother even offered to donate her kidney to me.

My mother's kidney was a perfect match. But as a schoolteacher, *Appa*'s income could not manage the unexpected high medical expenses. So, we sold our house for the transplant surgery. The expenses extended even post-transplant due to the many incidents of rejection that I faced. But the biopsy showed the kidney was fine. Then gradually, things settled down."

My co-passenger was sad and was nodding in agreement. Then he asked all of a sudden, "So how long ago was the transplant?"

"30 years yesterday," I said, thinking it was such a long time back. I remembered the day I had congratulated my 90-year-old mother and sought her blessings. Her golden words were, "30 years is okay, but I think you should aim for a lifetime. All our sacrifices must be worthwhile."

Suddenly, I saw that my co-passenger was fidgety. When I looked at him questioningly, he said, "My wife had a transplant last year. We want to have a kid. We are unsure if it is possible. Can you tell me how you managed to keep the kidney running for so long?"

I quickly assured him, "Having a kid is no problem. My son was born post my kidney transplant."

Then I shared my secrets. I knew it would help his wife.

I had to honour my mother's sacrifice. So, I became very strict with my eating habits and followed a *sattvic* (simple) lifestyle.

My day starts with meditation, something my wife is now wholly involved with, followed by a long morning walk. It is followed by a simple but wholesome breakfast. Lunch is a home-cooked meal, with less salt and low in spice. Evening tea is with biscuits. Meals are always eaten hot, and I stay away from instant food. I also avoid crowded places such as theatres.

After a few minutes of thinking, nodding and murmuring, he thanked me and got up to go for a wash.

Looking out of the window, I recalled how I formed a trust, the Kidney Foundation of India. Through the trust, I have been associated with many people to work towards helping subsidised dialysis.

But I knew there was much more to do. I simply had a long way to go, as the poet Robert Frost said.

On my trust and charity work – I spread my wings to conduct more awareness events in different parts of Kerala.

V G Chandrasekharan
Dialysis: some dialysis
Transplant: 30 years
Founder, Chairman, Kidney Foundation,
Secretary-General, Confederation of Charitable Organisations,
President, Federation of Organ Recipients Association &
E.C. Member, The Kidney Warriors Foundation
(One of India's longest surviving renal transplant recipient,
living 30 years with a donated kidney.)

GETTING ORGANISED WITH HEALTH

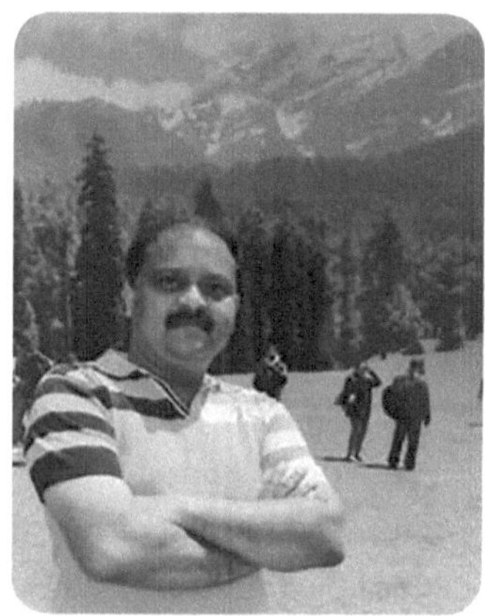

Diabetes

I really can't believe I reached this stage in life. Twenty years ago, in the results of a blood test, I was shocked to see my blood sugar levels higher than the permissible range. Immediately, I met our family doctor, who prescribed me the required dosage of insulin to maintain the functions of the pancreas. Some diet suggestions were given, which were followed as much as possible. The exact nature of the complication I could face was not known to me.

Life was fine. I believed my health was fine with the medication and the small diet changes. My work in the marketing field meant lots of travel. So, unknown to me, things were brewing deep within.

In 2011, I said goodbye to the job that compromised my health, and I became more conscious of my health and diet. Though I tried hard to curb my blood sugar, it was still high. In 2015, I was diagnosed with hypertension. The BP medicines did little to comfort me. Further tests revealed that the haemoglobin had gone down to 8.2 g/dl. So, I was advised pomegranate juice and iron capsules. When there was no improvement, I did a blood test to check for urea and creatinine.

Another shock! Creatinine had gone up since my last check-up 7 months ago. It was 1.9 mg/dl and now it fluctuates between 1.9 mg/dl to 2.1 mg/dl.

Life with such invisible diseases makes us very insecure. There's constant worry when one has such major kidney problems.

Rajesh Shrivastava

HOW FAR TO TRAVEL FOR DIALYSIS?

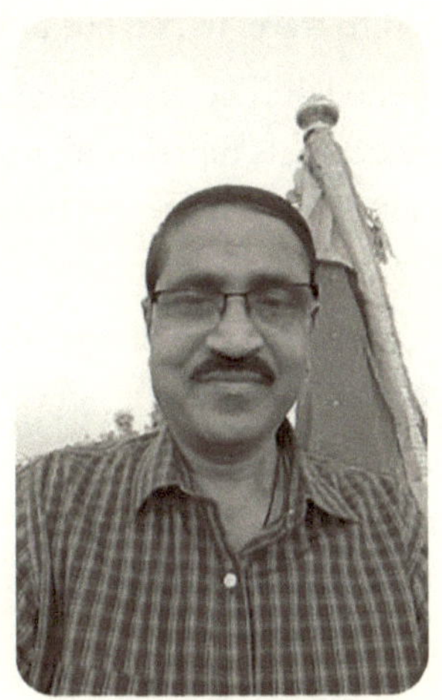

Hypertension

"Abhijit, let's go for lunch," someone called out to me, but I was too busy with work to even respond. This was a busy period in a government office as, in a few months, the 2013 state elections were to start. In the pre-election period, work multiplies. Moreover, I was also not hungry. For the past few days, I had felt a loss of appetite and nausea. This bothered me.

Then one day, I noticed swelling on my face and legs. My face was so swollen that my eyes looked funny. So, I went to my family doctor. Shocked to see my eyes slightly disfigured, the doctor began tests for paralysis. In the meantime, routine blood tests brought out the truth.

The biochemistry reports were fully highlighted by pathologists. It showed creatinine level was high at 4.4 mg/dl and all other constituents were also above the normal mark. The doctor quickly understood where the problem was. "It's not paralysis but a kidney failure. Please meet a nephrologist urgently." He was talking about a kidney failure and many things he said were like rocket science to me.

My mind was racing. *In Bollywood movies, they have kidney failures and transplants. This is not a movie. How can it be part of my life?*

Yavatmal in Maharashtra, with a population of over 130,000, is recognised for its agricultural produce. It is surrounded by many prominent districts—Amravati, Wardha, Chandrapur, Nanded, Hingoli and Washim—and has good potential for specialised medical services. A few years back, an airport had also been established, so emergency services could be handled. Hence, I was surprised to find that there was no nephrologist in the region. I had to travel to Nagpur to meet one.

A glance at the report was enough. The nephrologist straightaway broke the news that my kidneys had shrunk in size, so its functioning had reduced significantly. In due course, it could lead to CKD. He advised me to get hospitalised immediately to avoid further damage.

Assuring him that I would come back soon after the elections, I left. I was given medicines to maintain my health and reminded again of the need for dialysis. I nodded as if I was in full control of my life.

While returning to Yavatmal, I kept thinking, *After all, it is only dialysis. After the election, I will go and finish it. I have so much responsibility before the elections. I have no time to breathe.*

A reader would think, "How ignorant or negligent he was." Maybe I was a little of both. But I am sad and admit that due to this, I paid a very heavy price. Back home, I got very busy with the election work, without much thought about my health. My appetite was so bad that at some stage, I stopped eating altogether. I was overcome by dizziness and was perpetually with low energy. There was noticeable weight reduction. My health was sliding. I felt breathless, missed office on several occasions and felt embarrassed about my irresponsible attitude towards my official duty.

Finally, my family made a decision. I was admitted to a Nagpur hospital, where I was put on haemodialysis. In the 2 years of dialysis period, I tried many alternative treatments. These treatments made me sicker. One day, I got diagnosed with a lung infection with fluid. It became impossible for me to even take a step. I was rushed to Pune, where I got treated for the lung infection.

We decided to end the trauma and go ahead with a transplant. Thanks to Sarita, my life partner, whose kidney saved my life!

Though excited about the life-saving transplant, I was worried. It was my deep faith in God and love for my family members that made me overcome the hurdles that confronted me, so I could enjoy my new life.

After the transplant, I met many more challenges such as acute memory loss, ulcers on the abdomen, fungal infection and others. But life showed how trivial these were compared to the extreme hardships that I had already faced.

Now, it's a few years after the transplant. I'm absolutely fine, attending office every day, enjoying family life, engaging myself in divine and social events that give me peace.

I remember American politician Xavier Becerra's quote- "Individuals with kidney disease who are able to obtain treatment early experience a higher quality of life and are able to maintain more of their day-to-day activities, including keeping their jobs."

The healing power of God is working in me right now. Every day I get better.

As I look back, I wonder how other patients in Yavatmal and its neighbourhood could manage to travel like me to get treatment for kidney failure.

Though some dialysis facilities are there, more machines and better dialysis techniques need to be introduced. I hope, sometime soon, some efforts will be made to develop the region. People here may have the money for the treatment, but the lack of awareness and facilities are of far greater concern.

Abhijit Gavhankar
Transplant - 3 years

PEOPLE SAY, "IT'S A RICH MAN'S DISEASE"

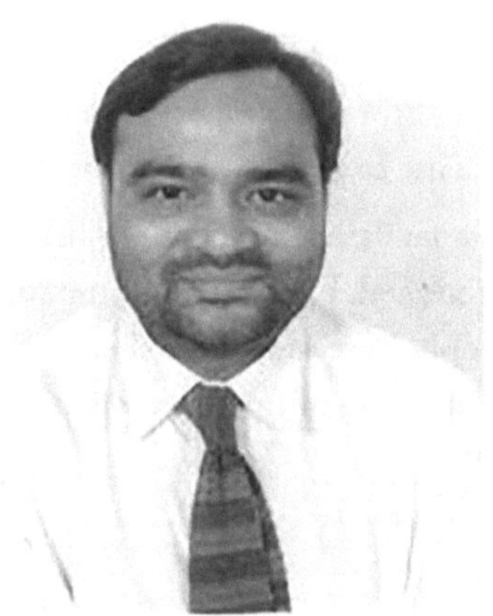

Hypertension

The flight was delayed by an hour. I let out a huge sigh. Another long wait, when I longed to be home to nurse my persistent headache. It was as if a hammer was hitting at my temple. *Last night's client meeting, those alcoholic drinks, the late dinner and the little sleep,* I grimaced.

Oh, a good night's sleep was just what I wanted. My hope for home-cooked food has vanished into thin air. I must recover from this hangover, were the thoughts running through my mind. Walking towards a less-populated area, I lit my second cigarette in half an hour. I really needed to relax.

Heading one of the world's most reputed consulting firms with offices in 6 cities meant a hectic work life involving travel and long hotel stays. The silver lining was having a personal trainer with whom I worked out each morning when I was at home in Mumbai.

Over the next few days, the headache became unbearable. I asked my secretary to seek an appointment with my family physician. The doctor checked my blood pressure and gave me some shocking news. My blood pressure was high, but fortunately, my stress tests were normal. Medications were started to curb the blood pressure.

I continued with my lifestyle; travel, business growth, smoking, reasonable drinking habits and the eating out associated with travel. Engrossed in work, I had little time to reflect on other matters, least of all my health, which the medicines were supposedly handling.

Things changed before the start of the new millennium. A casual visit to my physician in December revealed my BP was in the range of 180/110. The physician wanted to rule out the possibility of resistant hypertension.

After much persuasion, my family doctor got me to reluctantly agree to a random urine test. A trace of albumin was found. Consultations with a nephrologist confirmed it was proteinuria, (presence of albumin in the urine). A biopsy identified it was proliferative glomerular nephritis. The genesis could probably be rheumatoid arthritis, an autoimmune disease that probably was inherited from either or both paternal and maternal grandmothers.

Diet and medication to maintain the impaired kidney condition were started. However, by August 2000 I was ready for haemodialysis. On 21st October 2002, an unrelated donor offered me a kidney. What seemed a great new beginning grew into one of my worst nightmares. By January 2003, proteinuria had set in. A biopsy was conducted to confirm it. Within 10 months of my transplant, I faced a graft failure.

Quickly going back to haemodialysis got me thinking deeply. *Will this be my life, my future? The machine silently moving the red fluid in my body while I lie down like a moron,* I thought often.

Through such disturbing thoughts, some new pathways emerged. *I need to conquer the disease and be on top of it. Dialysis is a "D" that denoted depression, denial, diet restrictions, dependence and disruption. One by one these mental blocks need to be eliminated so I can lead a good quality life. There has to be some way,* I thought to myself.

I challenged myself to take the first step. With great foresight, I made fundamental changes to accommodate my new lifestyle.

Given that I would spend 3 ½ hours at the dialysis centre, I would need to employ this time effectively. 12 hours on dialysis was dedicated as my mini office time with the blackberry shooting off emails. So, clients servicing was never an issue. Music was good for my heartbeat, so I listened to soulful music while I read magazines and updated myself on engineering news around the world.

Slowly, depression was shown the door. Life was as much fun as I managed to make it. Saturday nights, bingeing with friends over drinks and dinner, and movie time was also featured. Vacation with dialysis was part of my annual calendar of events. So, I did not really deny myself life's pleasures that I was accustomed to. Diet restriction was well managed as I was in a happy mental state. I did not depend on anyone as I organised my financial affairs. My life went on without disruption and my wife could go back to work.

Gradually, I understood that business travels were difficult. I made a new strategy, which meant making a slimmer, more efficient organisation. Working over 48 hours a week on many large, reputed infrastructure projects in Maharashtra made this change worthwhile.

But more than that, I made my life's biggest statement:

3 Days on Dialysis, 7 Days of Life

With this slogan, I marched on with dialysis these past 17 years. There was no going back in time to ask, "Why did the transplant fail?"

I simply walked, head held high, and never lost focus on my objectives. I simply chose to make changes in my life to fit my dialysis in the scheme of things.

When I reflect on life, I clearly see the role my doctor played in encouraging me to do a simple urine test. Identifying the kidney disease early alerted me, the globetrotting businessman, to review my future professional plans.

Today, I'm a happy man, not held back, but on my front foot. I reiterate that kidney disease is a rich man's disease. Treatment is possible for the rich, who can become paupers, and the poor have no chance to live. This is definitely the case in economically developing countries where medical insurance does not cover the cost of treating chronic conditions.

I recall meeting a supervisor in 2004. The man was from Udaipur in Rajasthan, where only 1 dialysis unit was available and hence, he could not be treated. The fact is, however, that the number of people diagnosed, the number receiving treatment and the number of survivors cannot be estimated. The lucky survivors are only a handful.

I believe social workers are needed to help patients tide over emotional, financial and other issues.

Anand Dalal
Dialysis: 17 years
Transplant: 10 months

URINARY TRACT INFECTION LED TO CKD

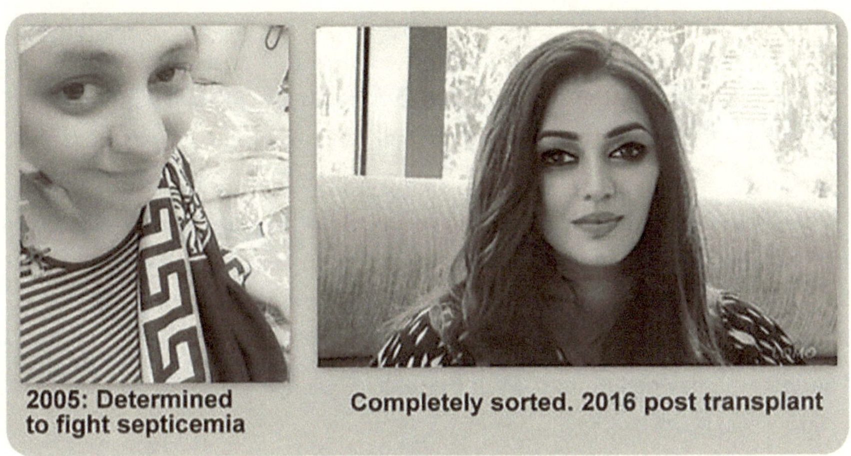

2005: Determined to fight septicemia

Completely sorted. 2016 post transplant

Urinary Tract Infections

"UTI – I mean urinary tract infections are common, Ms. Gita. Almost all people get it sometime, don't worry about it. Simply get these medicines, and you should be fine!" he gave a warm smile as he handed over the prescription and talked about general things to put my mind to rest.

Heaving a sigh of relief, I left the clinic, did some shopping, picked up medicines and started my 'treatment,' so to say.

Until June 2005, I had never experienced UTI, but now it became recurrent and these medicines brought out the worst in me. That's what I thought but very soon, my world seemed to crash. I was rushed to a medical emergency. I recall being wheeled into the ICU and also heard doctors saying, "Put her on the ventilator immediately." Thereafter, I was in a dark world.

For 2 months, I was in the ICU, though oblivious to my state of health. Due to an overdosage of medicines, I had septicaemia, in lay terms, blood poisoning and I was being treated. While on the ventilator, my family wrapped me with great love. My mother and sister were talking to me to awaken me, and on my mother's birthday, I actually squeezed her hand. These small things mean so much, I realise now.

By now, most parts of my body were ravaged and some organs were shutting down. The doctors took permission to administer some experimental medicines for septicaemia. There was a 50% chance of recovery.

My family was watching this drama, as tense as they could be. But they had to take chances. Slowly, the medicine awakened my body as if some magic potion was injected and my recovery process started. All but my kidneys, it seems.

I came out of my stupor to see myself hooked to a dialysis machine. In my 31 years (at that time) I never knew a thing about dialysis. I looked at the scary, menacing machine and seeing tubes with blood running in them, I was in a great shock. In an emergency situation, a catheter had been fitted, now they needed to fit a permanent one. I was very disturbed and cried through the 4 hours of dialysis, looking at the ceiling. All around me were many people hooked to machines, so it was really a sad time.

Then issues around my legs become very obvious. My legs were paralysed with 2 months of forced bed rest in a semi-conscious condition. So, there were physiotherapists helping me. Even things like pulling my body up to get into a sitting position with a rope tied to the end of the bed was so painful that I would cry.

Suddenly, it dawned on me, "Will I be able to walk, ever?"

"Was I destined to be like this?"

This very dark thought made me sit up and *'Do'* what I wanted to. Demolish the word *impossible.*

From where I got the strength, I never could understand, but that was the game changer. I designed my own therapy pattern. Though the physiotherapist felt I was not ready to put my feet on the ground, I told her, "Let me fall, I will get up and fall again, maybe."

As an afterthought, I added, "Please help me stand on the ground."

I can't explain what it felt like to put my feet on the ground. It was exhilarating. I took 3 to 4 steps and collapsed in a chair placed next to me.

From that day, I started walking, progressing from people supporting me to using a walker and then a walking stick. I promised myself, "By the end of this month, this walking stick will fly out of the window."

A friend asked me once, "Did you blame yourself or say, 'why me'?" I was surprised, but said simply, "No, I knew I'm the master of my own destiny. I have to move out of bed and into the wide world."

That statement made, I kept my promise.

From 2006–2015, I was not on dialysis. All the bad dialysis experiences were behind me. So, I charted my own plans to get better. Devised my diet with high-quality protein and managed to keep my potassium and phosphorus levels in check. It meant I had changed my lifestyle totally, be it my diet or other aspects of health.

To improve my health, I began working out at the gym and spin cycling, doing 2 sessions back to back. No way would I let the opportunity to survive slip by.

Was it a weak moment when my body gave up?

I was noticing the levels rising and though I dreaded and hated the thought, I needed haemodialysis in the last months of 2015. I hated it more than before. I cried; my body was too exhausted the next day post dialysis, so I became wheelchair friendly again. To remove myself from this rut, I chose peritoneal dialysis.

Again, a catheter in the abdomen needed to be fixed and I had to manage my own dialysis. 2-3 litres of dialysate solution dwelt in my abdomen doing the cleaning job. So, 4 times a day I would remove the fluid and replace it with fresh fluid. It gave me more flexibility for water and food. But I got some serious infections, requiring some treatments and surgeries.

Finally, God sent me a saviour. My darling sister agreed to donate, to be my live kidney donor.

24th January 2016 became my life's most memorable day. The transplant, done under a renowned doctor from Chennai, was a path-breaking concept developed by him with UK doctors, where one needs no steroids post-transplant. This was possible through the use of a drug called **Campath**.

I know my sister also faced some recovery issues for 2 months. Of course, even as I was recovering, I was unhappy seeing her struggle in pain. But both of us are now enjoying a normal life.

I can really breathe easy. I will never forget any of these past 12 years of my life. Tough as it was, it gave me a reason to talk about my troubles so that people in India can understand and take the right action.

I have been troubled by seeing the helplessness in the eyes of patients, more so of children undergoing dialysis.

I know for a fact that more organs are needed.

- **Family members coming forward to donate must definitely be considered as a rule.**

- **For a person whose family member has had an accident and is brain dead, please remember to donate organs. You will save 8 lives. Your sorrow will diminish as you see them live.**

- **Become more compassionate so you can feel happiness for others.**

The organ laws have made it difficult to even get a donor within a family. Family members see the process as harassment and think donating an organ is a criminal activity. Donors are our saviours. They need to be held in respect and not treated with suspicion.

I needed a lot of willpower. So, I know everyone will need that for fighting chronic kidney disease. Actually, they will need power with a good strategy to find survival.

My doctor gave me painful news when he asked me not to consider having a baby. All my maternal instincts were hurt as this came as a shock. How much I wanted to have babies. Today, I think it was the right advice. In fighting to survive, I may not have played a good mother. Neglecting a child is a great disrespect to humanity.

The transplant has put me on the road to happiness. I plan to surround myself with people who have love and compassion.

Gita Sagar Chopra
Dialysis - 1 year
Transplant - 2 years

VERY TAXING EMOTIONALLY WHEN IT IS GENETIC

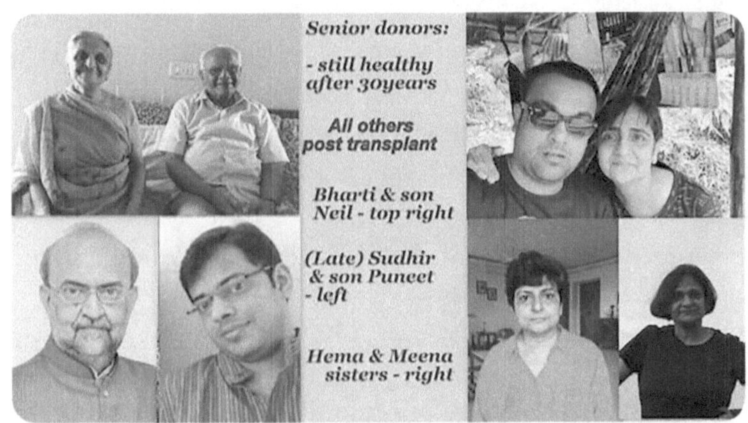

Glomerular Nephritis

The doorbell kept ringing. I was in a deep sleep and could hear the insistent ringing. Finally, with some effort, I dragged myself out of bed only to find Divya and Rohit at the door. Rohit's hand was poised on the bell, ready for his finger to press it for another long ring.

Sighing with relief, Rohit said, "Hey! What's up? Why aren't you answering either the door or the phone calls?"

I walked back into the room and slumped into a chair and said simply, "Hey... Sorry guys... What's the time?"

"It's lunchtime and we were waiting for you at subs. You know Divya! She was simply getting hyper."

I washed and dressed as soon as I could, and we left for lunch. I found the 10-minute walk to the university campus the most difficult walk of my life.

Breathless, I said with disgust, "I feel so weak that I can hardly move my legs."

This surprised Rohit, who said, "What are you saying? Yesterday you beat me in the basketball game. You are the sports guy, always wanting to get to the field. Now you are complaining!"

Divya glared as she added her observations, "You know what? You have been skipping meals. I have noticed at least on 3 occasions you were playing with your food."

Then after a moment, full of concern, she said, "Puneet, are you alright?"

I simply shrugged my shoulders and putting up my hands weakly I said, "Just chill, guys. There is no need to bring the roof down."

At 24 years, I was completely in control of my life. It was well planned when I entered Ohio's Wright State University to pursue my Masters in electrical engineering.

Yes, life had been good; I was enjoying my stay and my future career plans were just ahead in sight. So often I let my mind take me through the corridors of the corporate office. I would rub my hands in excitement and smile confidently. Life was just there at arms' length.

But today, I had no thoughts for anything. Definitely no thought for food! I wondered, "Am I really hungry?"

But during lunch, my lean contribution to the table talk drew attention from all around the table. I rubbed my legs as I admitted, "I'm sorry, guys, but I am feeling low; very weak."

Dropping everything else planned for the day, the group drove me to the university clinic.

As luck may have it, the doctor was a patient man. He heard me through and started examining me.

The first problem was high blood pressure at 170/110.

The doctor asked a quick question, "Are you on any blood pressure medications?"

"No, doctor. I'm not on any medicines."

Quickly, he authorised preliminary blood tests.

Tests revealed very low haemoglobin at 8.2 mg/dl (normal values: 13-18mg/dl).

More tests were needed, so I was admitted into emergency care. When the BP was checked again, it had shot to 210/160. They were worried that I could have internal bleeding. An ultrasound was done, and though I was anxious about the result, I had to wait in suspense the whole night. Next morning, the doctor informed me it was Chronic Kidney Failure.

The news left me shocked and seemed to make me numb. Even as Rohit and Divya were trying to comfort me, ridiculing the doctor and his competence, I could see the hospital corridors where I played as a kid, waiting for my mom to return. It was the time my father was seriously ill, in need of a new kidney.

That experience helped me now to see how my life would emerge in the days to come.

Slowly, all of it came back.

Stories of my aunts, my granddad and grand-uncle were often narrated in passing. I had hardly paid attention to minute details. Maybe I had fear?

I knew I had to make a call home, to my dad, a few hours later when India would wake up.

I didn't pause to think how dramatically my life would change.

The call to my parents came with multiple lines of conversations. Finally, it was decided. The US doctor spoke with our family nephrologist, Dr. B V Gandhi, who worked with all our family members. Nothing was new, but I had to swallow hard to suppress the hurt that the knowledge of kidney failure brought with it. It would simply tip the balance of my life from the safe zone to utter chaos. Suddenly, the edifice of a fantastic future came crashing down and lay at my feet, in a million particles of dust with little market value.

I returned to India to be treated by my family doctor. A few sessions of dialysis and thereafter, my mother donated her kidney. But I had to face another trial. The kidney did not kick in as well as expected, driving me down to the dialysis centre. In some time, another transplant became possible.

Through all this, as a young man, I watched my life move into an unpredictable state. Life was a serious business of health care. Memories of wonderful days from the past hounded me, but the stability attained now could never be compromised.

But with the right attitude and inspiration from the people around me, I collected my thoughts and created a niche for myself. I had chosen a career path and will emerge a star, leaving all constraints on the back burner. I will chase realistic dreams that keep me grounded while touching the peak of success.

I always felt my friends in the US were so marvellous. They took such good care of me and saw that I got treated. I also feel grateful for the doctor's early detection of my CKD. It was most timely.

My own view of life, after my experiencing so many unsure moments, is in a blog that I wrote some time back.

"Life's challenges are not supposed to paralyse you; they're supposed to help you discover who you are and get the best out of you."

- Puneet Gandhi

Overview

Glomerular nephritis has plagued several generations of my family. Though not always genetic, a trend was noticed in this interesting family. Whether there will ever be a full understanding about the onset of the disease is a matter of great debate, but such families will forever live in the fear of how the disease could impact future generations.

I was the 3rd generation to get the disease. Recently, my second cousin, Neil, Bharti auntie's son also had a transplant, giving us a loud and clear message that it can be carried down generations from the male (my grandfather → father → me) and female genes (my grand-uncle → his 3 daughters (of 4) → one daughter's son). And while my father, Late

Sudhir Gandhi, had glomerular nephritis, the disease escaped his brother, who was able to donate his kidney to my father when the first transplanted kidney failed.

However, my father's cousins—Hema, Bharti and recently, Meena—had the disease. One sister has escaped it. Or has she? It started with my grandfather and his brother.

The chance of someone not under the rudder is also a matter of speculation. Families face the fear and the suspense till everyone is tested and cleared from the threat of the disease.

In many families, the decision to marry and/or conceive may be governed by such unknown factors, which are beyond the realm of human control.

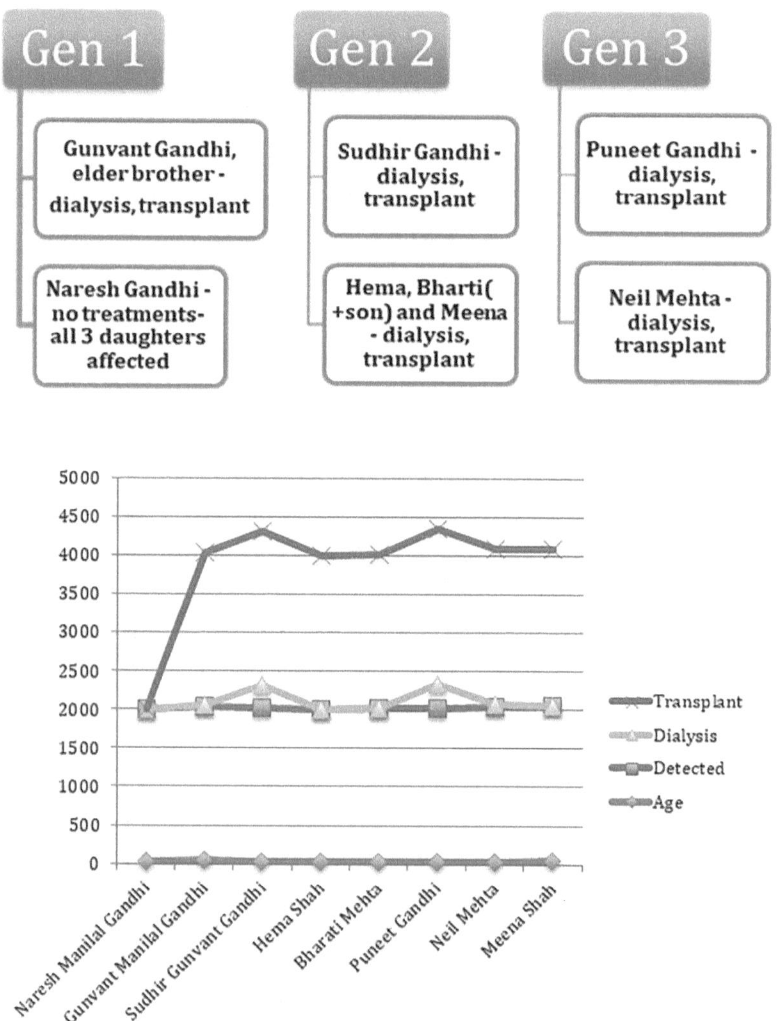

2 brothers: 2 familes with CKD (Total 8 members)

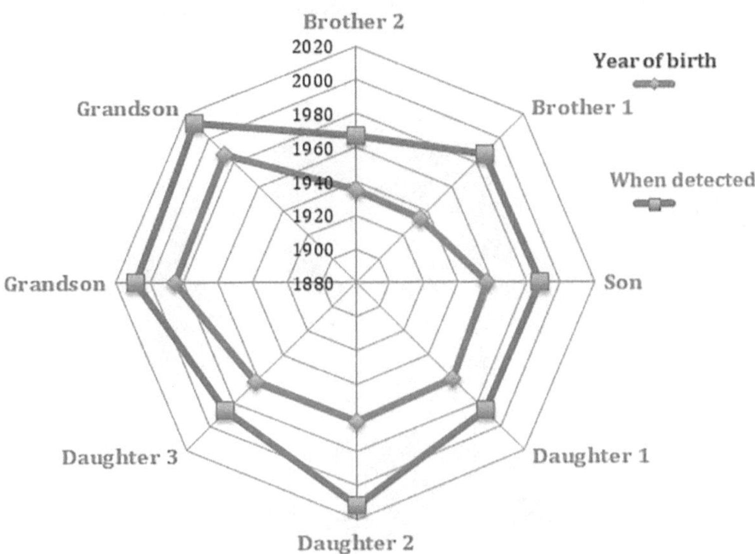

Observations

The mental strain caused by a single patient entering the various stages of the disease is huge, consuming every bit of energy and finances too. If this was repeated at different times with several family members, the mental toll will be humongous.

A commendable aspect of this particular case study is that, other than accepting the disease, this family understood their singular goal of survival. Interestingly, in providing treatments, members of the family were forthcoming to play the altruistic role of a donor, without a doubt. Such show of unity is very difficult to be replicated across other families under similar circumstances.

There's plenty of ongoing research. Some genetic studies may bring some results in less than a decade. Some great research will ensure that the disease ceases to be genetic and loses its power to transfer to the next generation.

Author's note: Late Sudhir Gandhi shared with me his continuous effort to bring down the cost of CKD medicines by convincing the Government to waive off duties on them.

DEFYING CKD AND CANCER

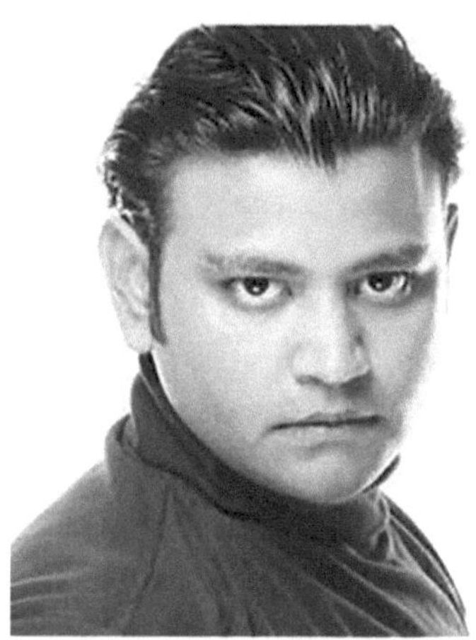

Kidney Cancer & CKD

"Don't ever come to me if you want to cry," she shouted, looking at me angrily. "I want to talk to people who want to fight."

I sat there stunned, shocked into silence. For a moment I wondered, "Why is she talking to me like that?" Silenced, a small moment of calm, I breathed, throwing a sly glance at her.

I know I should not lose control of my emotions, but what to do? I was one among the 2% of rare cases where a post-transplant drug's side effect caused cancer. I was now totally on the edge.

She offered me a glass of water. The cold water calmed my nerves. I began describing my long and winding journey with many episodes in the hospital. It's almost as if I was running a relay race. The baton was passed and I ran to another destination, but I was blindfolded and I ran endlessly to find my destination! I talked about how my kidney disease was diagnosed.

"In 2005, I was an aspiring 26-year-old trying to switch jobs. I went for medical tests to fulfil the pre-employment requirements of a job. I remember that evening; I was excited about the next day's interview when I collected the reports. But within a few minutes, I was shocked to read about traces of blood in my urine. The ultrasound talked of shrunken kidneys and the blood test showed high creatinine at 2.7 mg/dl. Later, when I met a nephrologist, I was advised a steroid treatment, apart from controlling my diet with low protein and salt.

Doubting the advice, I did an all-India trip, seeing doctors and confusing myself with many different treatments. By 2011, my creatinine had risen to 6.5 mg/dl without any symptoms. About this time, I also got married.

A friend introduced me to an ayurvedic doctor, known to have cured many patients. A week into medication, my creatinine shot up to 22 mg/dl and haemoglobin dropped to 5 g/l.

I began dialysis very soon, scheduling them in the early mornings so I could head straight to work afterward," I completed, so she knew my story.

"Oh, that *ayurvedh* probably wasn't even a certified *ayurvedh*," she said knowingly.

"You could not find any suitable donor?" she continued kindly, with real concern in her eyes.

"No, it was not possible. So, after starting dialysis, I got listed for a cadaver in Mumbai, Pune, Chennai and Ahmedabad. After a year and 9 months, I got that wonderful call. 5 people ahead of me on the waiting list refused the cadaver kidney, so I was allotted the kidney.

How fast things happened, I could hardly come to terms with the happy news. I was taken for the surgery by 9 am. By 5 pm, I recovered and my family was waiting in anticipation to see me wake up and talk. The good news was the new kidney made urine," I concluded.

My wife nodded as if in anticipation of more of the 'relay race' as I called it.

"The first 3 months passed blissfully but the problem started showing shortly afterward. In the 6th month post the transplant, I felt an intense pain in the abdomen. I was prescribed antacids, but when it didn't relieve the pain, some tests were suggested. The sonography showed a swelling, so I underwent a CT scan which confirmed huge ulcers in the small intestines," I continued.

I noticed my wife was hesitant when she said, "The doctors talked of a surgery. They spoke of it lightly."

"Now we are here because I'm just so scared. My wife wanted me to meet you."

We spoke about many things. She talked of some people who went through multiple organ failures and were without money for a transplant. Then she paused and added, "Rahul, you managed to come so far. Why? You have some courage to fight your way through and you also can financially manage treatments. Think if such a problem came to a person who was poor. What would have happened? God does choose people when he gives them problems."

I heard the lady talk. She didn't say anything that my friend couldn't say. It was not her choice of words, but the glint in her eye, the honest opinion said straight to my face and the gentleness of her voice. That was the magic and it worked.

I actually smiled and talked with her for 10 minutes about the date of the surgery and other details. I felt more confident to go ahead with the surgery.

I got admitted and was ready for whatever was to happen. Plenty of prayers were said for my successful return. But the real drama happened on the operating table when I was cut open and the doctors realised the ulcers could be something more. Surgery was paused and a sample was collected and sent for biopsy.

It was confirmed as lymphoma, a malignant cancer, with tumours ranging in size from 8-12 cm in size. The lymph nodes were removed. I was advised to be without water for a month; all food was in the form of supplements given intravenously. The anaesthesia affected the pancreas, pushing my blood sugar to 400 mg/dl. I was put on insulin to bring it down.

20 days later, I had to go back to the hospital for another operation. Till the surgery, I was not allowed to eat or drink through my mouth.

By now, my wife was shocked and speechless.

I spoke about how things had changed for me, "What had started slowly has grown big so fast. I had no time to relax. In just 6 years, I had to quit my job that I had worked hard to get and saw many dialysis patients succumb. It's tough, very tough to face the disease.

"But twice in my life, I prayed hard, asked God to take me away so my family did not suffer. Once when I was detected with CKD and now that I have lymphoma and need further treatment. But finally, my meeting with our mentor proved to be an extraordinary connection. Life changed and everything fell into place."

My wife was touched and she said, "You have the courage to face it all, but like your mentor said, we have no control over the events. Managing health with some yoga and spirituality will help."

I finished my 6 sessions of the 12-hour-long chemotherapy starting at 8 am. Though I was comfortable through the session, passing stools and urine were painful because of the uric acid in the medication. I had to drink 4 litres of water every day, which meant several visits to the toilet.

Before the 6th session, I had a high fever. This was a sign of more trouble. A chest X-ray and another scan showed more nodes. But the oncologist was unsure, so he arranged to conduct a bronchoscopy. He then did a surgery and collected a sample for testing. It was tuberculosis. So, there was another illness to attend to and treat.

After a year, a CT scan confirmed all was well. Now I needed to do an annual scan.

With a changed lifestyle, everything was managed well. Problems came and were resolved.

One day, I thought about my earlier years when I acted in plays. I had a circle of friends who were still engaged in theatre. I decided to get back to stage acting. It was my passion and being on stage gave me the power to express myself better, after having gone through many mind-blogging health experiences.

One fine day, I picked up the phone and called my friend who runs a drama company "Hi… Rahul Suprekar here. I know it's been a long time. I was in a play way back in 1996."

"Yes, will love to join your next programme!" After a pause, "Where shall I meet you? Okay. Thanks. I will see you."

The lights shone on me. I looked around as if searching for someone in the audience. Then in a loud and clear voice, I finished the last part of my act. "Life is going to be tough, always. If you keep fighting, victory is assured." I heard the thunderous applause and I walked off the stage as if I had conquered it all.

Rahul Suprekar
Dialysis: 1 year 9 months
Transplant: 4 years

30 YEARS OF OBLIVION

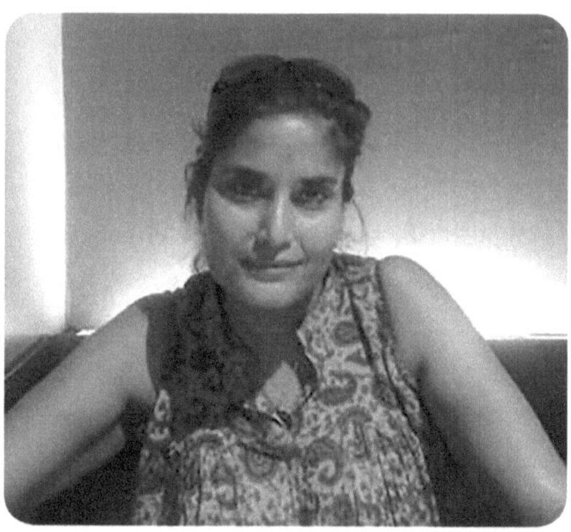

Hypertension

30 years of oblivion as I lived a life of discipline and restrictions, some that come with the territory after a transplant but mostly self-imposed! Both being the perfect balance to live life to the fullest. To reach this landmark, I cut myself away from the world of kidneys, worked to keep myself busy and productive. The only connection to kidney disease after my surgery has been the blood tests, reports and going to my nephrologists for my check-ups.

Flashback

At the time, I was diagnosed with renal failure, July 1986, there was a dearth of awareness and knowledge about kidney failure/transplant. Many, including us, didn't even know there was something called a renal failure and even if there was, it definitely did not happen to us or someone we knew, which lead to many a myth regarding the reason I had fallen ill, why specifically a renal failure leading to a transplant.

This, combined with how people's attitude towards me changed, pulled me back. It was either a look of pity, a look of "serves her right, she must have done something wrong" or asking my parents questions, which at most times didn't even relate to my illness. It bordered on pure gossip and smirks, so much so that it pushed me to a space where I went about the most normal life without discussing or talking about my illness. Even as I pen this, many do not have any idea about my transplant. It is time now to change some perspectives about how people perceive me and to comprehend the life of patients and their families who have to face the issues of kidney failure.

The Present

I hit the landmark of 50 years and I wanted to do something related to transplant. I went to the most logical person for a tête-à-tête; Dr. B. V. Gandhi, my nephrologist. Through his patient's family member, I got added me to a Facebook group, The Kidney Warriors. Reading all the posts, the information available, questions asked, the awareness of patients and their families put me in a shock - the world in this field had moved so much and so fast. It completely blew me away to speechlessness (a characteristic which is completely contrary to me). I was overwhelmed to find, unfortunately, not much had changed since I was diagnosed - the awareness regarding chronic kidney disease among the larger section of the society still remains obscure.

Embarking on this journey to create awareness, I am going to blog about my journey and experience dealing with the ailment, which continues to be clouded. A contribution not only to all individuals and their families to find their road to long-term well-being but to also applaud every individual and their family, who strive daily with such strength and faith.

Rita Patnaik
Transplant - 30 years

You may read her blog at this link:

https://beyoutheworldwilladjust.blogspot.in/2017/09/a-kickoff_22.html?m=1

ALWAYS AIM TO CONQUER

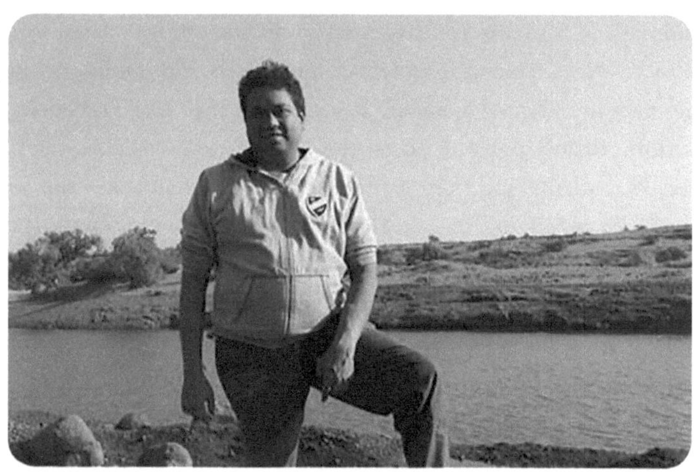

Hypertension

I was driving on the national highway. It was on one of my weekend trips to Pune on my teaching assignment. I saw the exit to Lonavala and smiled as I had when I had seen many such familiar signs during the drive. These were memory spots of my past. Memories of those precious moments that I treasure more than any wealth! I would pull them out during special 'alone' times to recall and re-live them. Sometimes I chose to share these anecdotes with people to whom it mattered.

I trek, even today, in those parts but to me, that trek was on recall even at the sight of a familiar bush, as if I had touched it every day of my life. The smell of the hills and the hour of triumph were sketched in my memory by some amazingly indelible stuff. I love to think about it every now and then.

The Western Ghats had beckoned me for treks in 1992 and the passion stayed with me for many, many years. My trekker friend group grew and 'V Hikerz' was formed. (Today, I lead a pack of 800 enthusiastic trekkers, as Mumbai's leading hiking group.) Through those years, I had explored and understood the hills very well. I was aware of those tricky spots, how to manoeuvre them and keep safe. And yes, that memorable last victory of a trek.

I smiled remembering how many friends, in all earnestness, had tried to dissuade me. They felt I could not do it with my reduced kidney function, with dialysis and the thumping fistula. But my love for challenges and the Bhimashanker trek had driven me to do the impossible.

Then, other incidents of the past surfaced without my intending to go there. It was about one of those treks. Very tiring and hectic but it was very enjoyable. There was a bit of rock climbing required, which meant I had to haul my body up using the strength of my arms. While doing this patch of the trek, a thorn got stuck in the base of my thumb and resulted in a swelling.

Once back home, I rested for a couple of days but the swollen thumb didn't become normal. I visited my family physician to get it examined. I was visiting him after a long time, so he was happy to see me. While chatting, he casually started examining my thumb and I could see the expression on his face change.

"The thumb is alright," he said. "But your pulse rate is extremely high. Let me measure your blood pressure." He made me lie down on his clinic bed. The readings were 190/130. "Very high," he continued. "You need to get hospitalised. This level of pressure is dangerous unless it is monitored closely." He also felt that I needed to stay away from work.

"That is tough," I told him. "As it is the month of March, my sales job involves maximising profits for my product category by the end of the financial year."

The doctor was firm and gave me little choice. Either I stay away from work for a few days, endangering my career or I take the risk and endanger my existence.

That was no choice really and I decided to rest. I could afford to lose out on my career right now and rebuild it later, but there was no point in endangering my life.

My mind went back to all the years of hard work. I had always been an independent person. My parents always encouraged me to be one. Since I passed out from school, I had given tuitions to school children and even paid for my college fees. After graduation, I worked for 2 years in an MNC bank to earn and save for an MBA.

I was good enough to get into MBA at NMIMS (one of the top 10 institutes in the country) in the 1ˢᵗ list in the open category. Post MBA, our batch was slightly unlucky as there was a recession and jobs were few. But I got into a top B2B company and worked hard to build a sales portfolio of around Rs 25 crore.

It involved a lot of effort. There were times when I would travel for more than 15 days a month. Food and sleep timings were erratic. Though we were put up in top hotels, the work involved travelling to factory locations in *mofussil* areas. Hence, there were a lot of times when we had to eat food from roadside *dhabas*.

In addition to this, I was very active socially. My community has a very active socio-cultural organisation, where I was secretary for 4 years, with annual elections. As part of this responsibility, I was in touch with the top musicians of India, organising their concerts and events. I had a really busy life. I guess a bit too busy for my body and it was now showing.

I rested for a few days and kept monitoring my BP. However, it showed no signs of coming down, so I underwent some more investigations. My creatinine was high and it meant that there was a problem in the functioning of my kidney.

Due to a BP of 160/140, doctors suggested I get admitted to a hospital for investigations, so I was hospitalised. A few tests were done. The only report that showed abnormality was the biopsy, which showed I had MPGN progressing to sclerosis. This was a dangerous situation. It meant I would go on dialysis very soon.

Not only that, I was told my activity levels would go down and worst of all,

I would have to give up trekking. Well, that meant I would need to change my personality. Something inside me was revolting.

Even though I was on leave, my colleagues from office kept calling me. When discharged from the hospital, I went back to work. Subtle hints were made on my illness, suggesting I might not be able to handle stress. Then it came as a blow when the management informed me that they didn't have any other vacant position to offer me.

I signed out and decided I would start my own advertising agency. But my 1ˢᵗ priority was my health, which was looming large, with a future possibly on dialysis.

I decided to try naturopathy. Anandashram is my 2ⁿᵈ home. I had been visiting the place since I could recall. The head of the ashram, Swami Satchidananda, asked me to come over and stay for a few days.

We started naturopathy treatment there. A strict diet with herbal juices, along with treatments such as sunbath, spine bath, etc. and I was feeling much better.

Slowly, the creatinine readings started improving till they came to normal.

I lived there for around 3 months. When I returned, I started my own advertising agency as planned. I was working with freelance designers though I did the visualisation myself. I was following the naturopathy diet and other treatment as well. The readings were stable. I was feeling far better.

My agency was also doing fine. I was working at my own pace, without too much exertion. I had done some work with 3 top brands and repeat business was also coming in. My dream of running my own agency was in a way getting fulfilled.

Then one day, I woke up to reality, rudely.

I had a bad fall at a Mumbai station and injured my back. I had a fever for more than a week along with a bad muscle spasm and by the time I recovered, my creatinine was more than 9.

It was too late to even go back to the ashram for naturopathy as the readings meant I had to start dialysis immediately. I underwent an urgent fistula surgery. During the surgery, my mind was disturbed again. I needed strength to face the situation.

I returned home after fistula and then went into a state of silence (*Maun Vrat*) for 3 days. These 3 days were filled with intense prayer and meditation, after which I was ready to face anything.

Luckily, by the time I started dialysis, my fistula was matured and ready for use, so I didn't need to use a catheter.

A new journey had started. Doctors told me I could not trek ever again and that I would need to curb my activities. Dialysis meant I would have to take concessions from work and therefore, my career growth hit a huge roadblock. But the appetite to win was not lost. I wanted to win against all odds; to win against people who had normal health, whose kidneys were working fine, who were passing urine normally.

I continued my agency work. Now I did more good work with top brands. But due to the cost of dialysis, I was unable to take my operations to the next level, where I could have my own employees and office.

I also wanted to do something for the kidney fraternity. I made presentations to kidney organisations like ZTCC on campaign ideas to popularise cadaver donations.

I finally got an opportunity to design a logo for ZTCC Mumbai. Seeing it in use even today, I feel a great satisfaction that they valued my creation even though it was for a token fee.

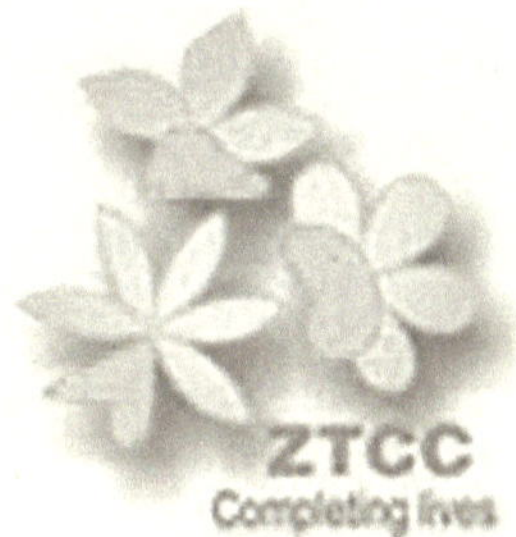

Around this time, in my haste to take my business to the next level, I started taking printing jobs. Printing has more margins than just creative designing and I thought that this would enable me to rent office space and start employing people. But I made a mistake. There was a printing error and I lost a lot of money. Yes, I realised that printing was a double-edged sword.

I went out of business. I had to take money from my parents for the 1ˢᵗ time in so many years, but I didn't have a choice.

This went on for around a year when some friends suggested I use my experience and knowledge to consult smaller companies in the area of marketing strategy.

In this free time, I had become comfortable on social media and had built a new network for myself. We had started going on short outings and enjoying ourselves.

One day, we went on a short trek and I felt I could really attempt serious trekking again. I thought, "No way, I am staying away from trekking… I need to be alive and live well too."

I began trekking more regularly. One of the treks that I could not go on was at Bhimashankar. I was feeling unwell and had to drop out at the last moment. Bhimashankar was one of my favourite treks and I really wanted to do it badly.

After the trek, my friends were happy that I could not join them. They felt that in certain places it involved hauling oneself up with our arms and I might not have been able to do it due to the fistula in my hand. My memories went back to the last trek before my kidney ailment was diagnosed. I felt dejected. Maybe I would never really be able to do all those beautiful treks again

Meanwhile, one of the meetings for consulting went off well and I was offered a full-time job. Since I was in dire need of money, I took it up. This was a very junior level and I took it up as I was unsure whether my body would be able to take the rigour of a full-time job.

As I had tested HCV positive at a centre where low-cost dialysis was offered, I shifted my hospital by then. Luckily, this hospital had a 24-hour-dialysis centre. I opted for late evening dialysis so that I could perform my duties at my full-time job without having to ask for concessions.

This was in the field of digital marketing. I picked up well. I was able to perform and my roles in the organisation started getting upgraded from just client servicing to key account management to business development and strategy, with the additional responsibility of public relations.

At the same time, I made new friends in the organisation and coaxed few of them to trek with me. After a few treks, I suggested Bhimashankar. I knew it would be a challenge for me. I also had it at the back of my mind that some friends had suggested I might never be able to do it, ever.

The group was small. I sort of mentally prepared them on what could be done in case there was a problem. I was the only one who knew the route well.

After late night dialysis on Friday, we worked on Saturday and left that evening. We travelled to Karjat, spent the night at Karjat station and went to Khandas (the base point for the Bhimashankar trek) early in the morning.

After a short prayer to the Lord, we started the trek. The mighty Bhimashankar beckoned me. The beauty of the place is really pristine in the monsoons with flowing streams, greenery all around, dense jungle and some breath-taking valley sightings. The waterfalls on the way are like the icing on the cake.

My friends were a great support. There were times we needed to take a break and we all did it together. At the point where my other friends felt I would not be able to cope, I did it easily. But in the last stretch (Bhimashankar needs a lot of endurance), I did feel like giving up. But we were in such a place that it was more of a distance to turn back and it was really a better idea to complete the trek. We took a longer than usual break and had some tea prepared by villagers.

Finally, we completed the trek in 6 hours. Earlier, I could complete the same trek in 4.5 hours. I requested my friends to excuse me for a moment. It was a very private, emotional moment for me. I cried. Almost inconsolably!

So what if it took longer? I had completed the trek. I had worked my way through areas where I had to haul myself up. I had done this after working a full day, performing in my role as a business strategist and competing with normal professionals whose kidneys were working fine. I had done this when some friends told me I would never be able to do it.

And then it was the moment, the moment when I reached the top. I managed to conquer the formidable peak, and yes, I had done it despite my fistula and being on dialysis.

"I did it!" my mind shouted.

It was just one of those treks. Very tiring and hectic but one that was most enjoyable! It put me on a new high!

Life had come full circle.

Samiir Halady is now the head of a digital agency and is currently a consultant in the area of digital marketing strategy. He is also working on a venture in rural tourism.

He is a keen photographer and makes his tourism as well as hiking trips memorable.

Samiir Halady
Dialysis: 17 years

FORCED TO LEAVE A FARMER'S LIFE

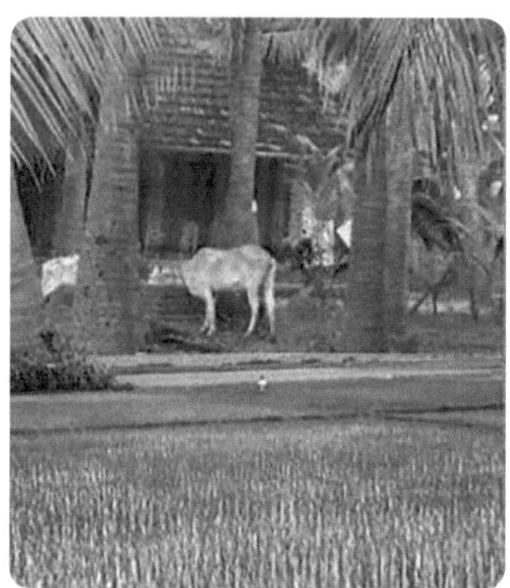

Hypertension

I turned back to see the lush green farms ready for a harvest. "Good crop this year," was my thought as I turned to look at my wife. Her eyes were swollen due to crying the whole night through. I could sense her sadness and anger. I chose to remain silent, trying to ignore and forget that I was also deeply hurt. I would be leaving the farm now and may never return. My life was so uncertain and my future was bleak.

In a short time, life had taken more than a 360° turn; a farmer was forced to leave his career as a farmer. I looked at my hands. They had worked on the soil, the seeds, the manure and irrigation. These hands had tilled the land at dawn.

I had lost everything in a single stroke. Apart from leaving the farm, I carried the burden of an unknown future and will see tomorrow's daybreak alone, estranged from a large family of brothers and their families. I will be walking among a population of so many scores of people, none of them known to me.

It had started with a swelling in my legs. The village doctor exclaimed loudly, making me jump, "Oh my god! Your blood pressure is very high. I think your kidneys are damaged." After a blood pressure check-up, he continued, "Most probably it is a kidney failure. Go see a specialist."

In a state of panic, I rushed to Mumbai to meet a nephrologist. After a blood test, he explained about my health and said, "Your creatinine is very high. It looks like your kidneys are not working."

When I returned home, I spoke with my family over our morning cup of tea. My elder brother looked at me silently. He then threw his towel over his shoulder and walked away without a word. I turned to look at my other brother. He cleared his throat and rushed to another room as if he remembered something important. As the day progressed, my wife and I saw everyone's attitude towards us change. It was as if I was infected with a contagious disease. My family's reaction was alarming. In the days that followed, things grew worse. I was a stranger, an unwanted person in my own house.

The tension finally snapped when I spoke of a transplant.

"You know we don't have money for a transplant!" said my eldest brother to break the silence and stop me from saying more.

Another brother commented, "It is a very expensive disease. Only a rich man can survive such a disease."

"You know," my elder brother continued, "people die with a transplant. It is not safe."

And after that, all conversation stopped. Total silence. It was as if I was not even there, standing under the same roof, eating dinner with them. No one looked at me. In the kitchen, the women ignored my wife. Realising that the financial drain of the disease was the family's biggest concern, I suffered silently as I knew no one would help me. I saw that my family members had deserted me when I was facing such a great challenge in life.

Things grew worse with each passing day. Then, with a heavy heart, I chose to leave the farm, leave my home, to forget that I was part owner of that ancestral property and that farming was my livelihood and it was so close to my heart. I knew I had to choose to get well and live.

I turned back one last time and said a quiet goodbye. I thought of my childhood. Running around the village with other kids, working on the farm, breathing the freshness of the farm air. My parents loved me so much. How much I will miss the familiar sounds of the cattle mooing or the hens kicking the dust! Everything will soon become a memory as if it was from another time and slowly dim away, forgotten forever. But inside me, the pain of being rejected by my family will take a long while to die.

I began dialysis at a facility in Mumbai at special rates for low-income groups. My wife offered to donate, but her kidney was not a match. The doctors advised me to participate in a swap transplant programme and I managed to receive a well-matched kidney. My wife's brothers were very supportive. They paid for the surgery partly and arranged to raise funds through charities and many individuals in Mumbai city.

Sangram Singh
Transplant - 5 years

Reflections: In his fight for survival, I saw a self-respecting farmer's life change suddenly due to a kidney disease. He was deprived of his humble farm life but was given a new working kidney. I'm happy he got saved but wonder about his mental state. He is now unemployed in the streets of a harsh city life in Mumbai, completely dependent on others for medicines and livelihood.

How will a farmer ever learn to live in a city? His only skill is farming; growing crops, watching the skies change their colour to dark grey to announce rain and look forward to a good crop season. How will an uneducated man meet this great challenge in life?

Someday, I hope he will find an occupation in the city so that he can truly survive, with a working kidney and happy disposition.

KIDNEY DISEASE, A GAME CHANGER

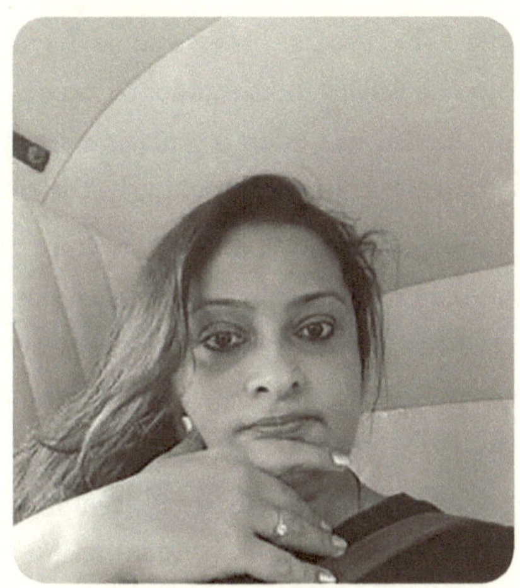

Hypertension

When a kidney fails suddenly, one speculates about the cause. At the age of 22, mine was due to the slow and silent killer, blood pressure. After 3 months of dialysis, my sister donated her kidney. My mother was happy that her children bonded to overcome a life-threatening disease. She took great care of us through the period and was a pillar of great support.

I was recovering well and nurturing my new organ.

But in some time, I got a whiff of other major life-changing problems brewing in our household. It seemed that overnight, my father's business, worth multi-million-pounds, faced an unexpected turbulence. Anxiety was riding high in the household as the storm could not be easily quelled. Each day new problems cropped up. Through this phase, my mother was keeping her eye on my health, but I sensed her real worry was in keeping the medicines flowing.

At odd times, she would ask, "Sejal, do you need to buy medicines?"

Taking a cue from her questions, I started saving medicines so that the stock could stretch over a longer period. In the eye of the storm, our own senses are sometimes dimmed. And very soon, the results of my action surfaced. It started with one problem and spiralled to another. Somewhere down the line, I lost my hearing and even the most sophisticated hearing aid could not fix it.

Anxiety due to all my health issues, along with the financial strain, caused my mother great turmoil. Internally crying, her health started to deteriorate and in some time, she left us orphaned.

The final nail was driven when the kidney was rejected. I can't even explain what the family faced at this juncture. It was a deep sense of loss and hopelessness.

The doctor agreed that I deserved another chance. My father was tested and the cross-match was negative, so he was found suitable to donate his kidney. However, due to my high sensitisation, I needed to undergo a plasmapheresis. The day prior to the transplant, another cross-match was done. Shockingly, the result was positive.

The news was devastating and it proved to be one that made my father, who was fighting against all odds to save me, lose his battle. To any bystander, it may seem like he took an easy way out, but his suicide was the greatest testimony to the forbearance of a man who fought to survive against so many odds. His daughter's kidney disease would not let him live peacefully.

I know in my heart that my greatest tragedy is not my affair with the kidney disease but the loss of my loving parents who were unfailing in their undying love and support.

At 39 years, I am waiting for a 2nd transplant for the last 6 years.

Sejal Jobanputra
Dialysis: some
Transplant: 4 years
Dialysis: 10 years

THROUGH CHILDHOOD WITH CKD

Hypodysplastic Kidneys

My 18 years of life with chronic kidney disease has taught me and allowed me to witness a beautiful concept of strength.

From the age of 7, I made multiple visits to the doctor. The clinic became walls of assurance to me. Every needle pricking me for blood test became a motivating factor for me to move forward. The medicines, in its literal sense, became life-saving. It was the combined effort and hard work of the doctors, the unwavering support of my family and friends and the absolute dedication of my mind as well as body that permitted me to have a kidney transplant on 17th February 2017.

Before the transplant, I strongly believed in rebirth, so I accepted the surgery as an opportunity to find a new life, with such a great courage that I never believed was in me. It almost felt like I had the will to resurrect and renew my kidney and this thought has kept me going.

I have come to understand that my health is what should come first. I have several people to thank. My mom, for being prepared from the very moment she heard about the transplant, staying steadfast in her purpose and keeping her health in proper condition. My father stayed with me day and night, next to my hospital bed, awake at odd hours and staying away from home. I have grown closer to him in those days and I wouldn't exchange them for anything. My *dada* and *dadi* always accepted and understood my conditions. They would sneak in sweets and chocolates so that I never missed out on anything during my childhood. Lastly, and most importantly, my doctor, for never giving up on me and guiding me through this journey and making this new life possible for me.

Having said this, my only hope is that I can motivate more people and gain inspiration from others, who in spite of their health condition have fought to survive and made their life.

Varnaya Sanghvi,
Transplant - 1 year

SAGA OF REJECTIONS

Hypertension

I remember that day very vividly. It was a day when my glowing life turned into a nightmare. As you know, some clocks can never be reset.

So, on this life-changing day, I had walked out of the pharmacy with the new blood pressure pills- *Posecar* manufactured by Roche Pharmaceuticals. This was recommended by my US doctor to stabilize my blood pressure. Of late my BP was behaving erratically. I had thought, "If this works for me… life will be peaceful again."

Back in India I had settled down to busy life with my law practice. Neck deep in work, I managed to keep my medical regime and life moved on. The lab reports had begun showing cyclosporine toxicity so the dosage was gradually reduced. But things changed in few months, when the lab reports showed a gradual rise in creatinine. It soon manifested in some discomfort that I began experiencing. In a quiet moment I shared my concerns with my wife.

For a long time Kalindi, would narrate the situation we had faced in 1993 as the most poignant moment in our life. But with kidney disease, each day we add our own unsure moment of being on the verge of death, till life swings back.

So my tryst with kidney disease started in 1993. I was 34 years then. My creatinine was astoundingly high at 21mg/dl with BUN at 400g/dl. It was shocking that I was still looking almost normal when a time bomb was ticking inside me. The cause was not detected; but doctors speculated it to be due drug related allergy.

Reality was, my life had gone for a toss with the chronic kidney failure.

Medical treatment in Mumbai had beckoned me from Delhi, where I moved lock stock barrel with my lovely family and my law practice. I was put on dialysis, but soon help came from my 63 year- old mother who was emotionally disturbed with my sudden illness. Without hesitation she stepped forward saying as gently as possible, "Let me give you my kidney. You are young and you have to take care of your wife and kids. I have heard that people can live even with a single kidney." Her persistence helped and within 6 weeks her kidney was transplanted.

My life had become wonderful again. My work kept me happy and my family life bounced back to a normalcy. Bringing some changes in lifestyle, I limited smoking and alcohol consumption.

So Kalindi was also concerned that after a successful transplant, the creatinine was rising. Without much loss of time anti-rejection treatment was started. But sadly my mother's gifted kidney was compromised and the medication didn't restore it.

Taking the setback in my stride and going back on dialysis was about the only option open to me. Some investigation on the new medicine *Posecar* unearthed some facts. It reacted adversely with cyclosporine. So when the dosage was reduced the kidney was rejected. Some time later, I heard that the drug was withdrawn from the market since many patients were gravely affected by its side effects.

Undeterred, I had gone for a second and third transplant. One rejected following a perforated intestine. Understanding the gravity I vowed never again, only to seize the next opportunity when it presented itself. It was a cadaver. But alas each kidney comes with its own destiny.

So today, I'm on dialysis for eleven years. I'm fine, remain active, keep busy with my practice and travel too. I enjoy an occasional drink, and do some exercise- swimming or going for ambles rather than walks.

All my kidney escapades have left their indelible mark, but I have no regret on where life has taken me. Years back, it hurt me to be the cause of grief to my wife. All her aspirations of finding a career as an economist were crushed long time back. Kalindi's steadfast support acted as my armor of courage through our worst times.

As for the woman who gave me a second chance, my mother, at 86 years is happy to still play golf and travel. So you see donating a kidney does not affect one's lifestyle.

As I sum up my life as a kidney patient, I see it spiked with lots of humor. Somehow blessed several times over, with a kidney, a transplant done but the goodbye to the kidney coming too soon thereafter, causing so much pain and agony, has to have a flip side. For all those kidneys that entered my body it could have been an "amusement challenge" on who could stay longest! They would have mocked me for my challenging them to stay on till end of my life.

But providence has been kind enough to make me a winner each time.

All my wife's prayers and the glint of hope in those tired eyes of the aged in my household were not wasted. I am truly blessed to be alive.

Vikram Philip
Dialysis : 19 years

KEEN ADVOCATE FOR SPREADING AWARENESS

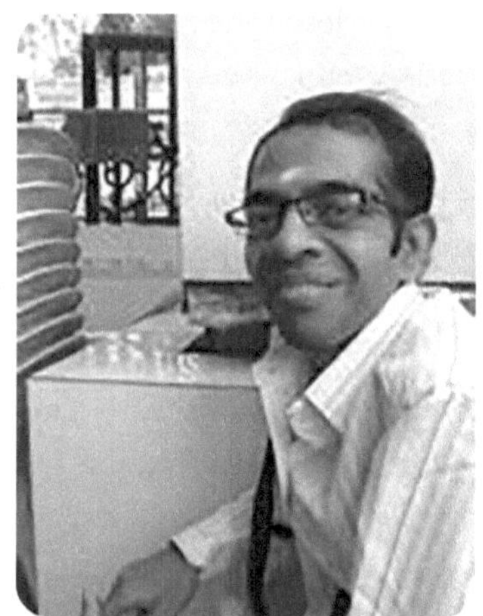

Glomerular Nephritis

I recall that first moment. *Dadaji* came out from the washroom and said what seemed a random statement, "One of you used the toilet and forgot to flush!"

I looked up distractedly, "Sorry *Dadaji*, I forgot but I was halfway through something."

Walking to me, he gently placed his hand on my shoulder and said, "*Beta*, did you see the foam in your urine?"

"Yes, *Dadaji*… there … It has always been like that… at least for some time now!"

"Okay, finish your studies. After your exams, we will go to a doctor to get it checked."

And then, when we went to the doctor, the whole truth surfaced.

March 1995 was the month that changed my life. The doctor asked for a blood test and a routine urine test. Next morning, we were able to do the tests and later in the day, at the doctor's clinic, we knew the truth.

"Sadly, Vishal has inherited his mother's illness. His albumin levels are a little high. The froth is, in fact, showing the presence of protein in his urine."

"*Amma* also died of the disease," I thought sadly, even as the emotion was choking me. "The albumin in my urine helped in tracking the disease."

For treating it, I was prescribed prednisolone, an ace inhibitor, and a few other medicines. As a young man, facing this grave disease was very tough. I was forever thinking of how my mother had succumbed to the disease and was a little troubled that my father, living in Canada, could only be reached sometimes over the phone. I began to feel lonely and was fighting the many emotions that filled me with deep anxiety.

Months later, a 2nd opinion confirmed the initial diagnosis. Some dietary changes were introduced and a biopsy was also suggested. But I could not go through it all. At odd moments, I was left confused. Sometimes the fear overtook my determination to get treated and then the overriding feeling was that of denial. I tried to find solace in the justification that I did not have the diseases because I did not feel any side effects.

Taking a firm decision to divert my attention to other aspects of life, I concentrated on my education. I shrugged off every conversation about undergoing further tests for the disease.

I graduated in microbiology and biochemistry. I felt good and worthy.

I would be lying if I say that I had forgotten about my simmering health issues, it was just that I refused to give it any credence. So, all in all, I basked in the glory of my graduation, at the cost of ignoring my health.

Sometime in mid-2000, I began noticing the face of change.

A blood test revealed my creatinine had spiked too high. I was hospitalised for emergency treatment and in November 2000, I had my 1st dialysis. As I went through my dialysis, sadness overcame me. I felt that the world had grown very small, as if I lived there alone, by myself. My twin brother, Brijesh, understood my feelings and tried to cheer me up.

And then came this extraordinary opportunity. 7 years after I started dialysis, my uncle offered me a kidney. I was overjoyed. I did not know how to control this overflowing happiness. Soon after that, the great day came. I got the kidney.

But fate had something else planned for me. The kidney gave me more problems than I could have ever imagined. I had heard stories of successful transplants and the doctors had assured me. But I wondered, "Why is the journey with my new kidney such a bumpy ride? Why is it not kick-starting despite all the attempts by doctors?"

Till then, my life revolved around my grandparents and Brijesh, but when I was in the hospital, fighting to hold the kidney, I missed my mother more than I ever did in all my 19 years.

Her void was felt at this juncture when a working kidney would give me a life of freedom. If only she was there, her presence and a small warm hug would have made me fight harder. This kidney going away was a huge loss. Life would never be the same. I will be back on dialysis.

Finally, I had to face that moment when I had to take my life's major decision. My heart cried, trying to hold on to that kidney and asking it to sit quietly. I looked out of the hospital window, watching the sunset, and decided, "Let the sun set, but I will live my life without misery, head held high." So, my moments of 'happy times' lasted for 7 months. I walked out of the hospital with every attempt to overcome my loss. It took time. But I lived through it.

My mother was missed many other times. I wanted to work, to be able to earn and pay for my dialysis. She could have motivated and put me on track. But Brijesh never let me down. He would say, "This is ours, not your battle alone. I'll work and you'll take care of your health."

So, as strong as the bond was between the twin brothers Ronald, who donated his kidney to Richard Herrick, creating the record of first successful transplant in Boston in 1954, we twin brothers bonded at an emotional level, far different and yet equally strongly linked for life.

Now on dialysis for 17 years, with 4 days of dialysis, I have changed in many ways. I keep a close watch on medicines, injections and medical follow-up as there is no room for compromise. Gradually, I developed a spiritual and philosophical outlook. Some evenings, I attend *bhajan* sessions at a community centre, which gives me great solace. It helps me strengthen my resolve to accept all situations positively.

Managing to live on dialysis meant embracing a lifestyle with limitations, as suggested by dieticians. I got involved in mastering my culinary skills and participated in diet competitions held by the Narmada Kidney Foundation. My recipes were appreciated and I won several awards.

On Facebook, I manage a support group, Milestone in Dialysis, with over 500 members who are on dialysis. Our group is interactive, with members sharing information and offering guidance to Indian as well as foreign patients. To understand the problems faced by patients, I interviewed many patients with video recordings. This brought in an appreciation of many unknown issues faced by them that changed my own feelings about why greater awareness is needed.

I'm keen on evolving new ways to cook for patients. I wish to occupy myself with activities related to diet and recipes for kidney patients.

Facebook brought me closer to new acquaintances and new friends. We came together to form a group proudly called The Kidney Warriors. Apart from online

counselling to patients and caregivers, we have started educating people about kidney diseases through events.

A diet book for dialysis patients is under development. The book is designed from a kidney patient's perspective, with my involvement at all the stages to make it the best renal diet resource for Indians.

I follow the dictum, "Always be happy and accept whatever comes, for they are the yardsticks for measuring one's inner strength."

Vishal Gadhia
Dialysis: 7 years
Transplant some months
Dialysis: 10 years

A COUPLE WIRED BY TELEPATHY

Diabetes

07.46 -7th Dec 2017: via Facebook messenger

I'm a kidney warrior. I have been on dialysis the last 2 ½ years. When you struggle with your life, your family also struggles. A strong relationship is built when we choose to love each other in those critical times when one is fighting to survive.

When I see my wife sharing not only my health problems but also taking care of my family's responsibilities, I realise how lucky I've been in finding such a perfect partner with whom I'm able to spend my life.

I think, besides medical treatment, one also needs family's affection. Wishing everyone good health and good luck.

Gurmeet Singh

08.22 -7th Dec 2017: via WhatsApp

My husband is on dialysis the last 2 ½ years. I took two words from the dictionary of life - Patience and Courage. The circumstances we ask God to change are often the circumstances God is using to change us. I feel responsibilities have no limit.

Life has put me in difficult situations but I never give up. Day by day, my smile increases along with my responsibilities. My life is not a battle. I am not going to fight or achieve any goal. I just want to serve humanity till the end of my end. May God bless everyone with good health and happiness!

Mrs. Karamjeet Kaur Saini

MARRIAGE GETS ROCKED

Hypertension

"How can she come into our home with kidney failure? This is surely a clever ploy to cheat us!" she shouted with vehement hatred. She went on with, "Her father and mother have schemed against us to cheat us!"

These words penetrated through my head even as I was trying to find the answer to the burning question, "How did I get kidney failure?"

One may say figuratively, the sounds of the shehnai had barely died and the colour of *mehendi* was still faintly visible when my marriage faced an unexpected turn.

I was married in the month of January. I can say it was the happiest day for my family. There was so much joy. I was excited to find the man of my dreams. He was handsome, well-placed in life and made me feel so good. My parents opened their treasure chest and gifted me handsomely. After all, marriage is a one-time affair in a normal household.

Slowly, I settled down into my new home and life with my husband and his parents. New home with some adjustments were all expected and I did my best to live up to my expectations of creating for myself a stable family life.

I remember that day in February vividly. Actually, that day has been inked in my mind as if it can never be wiped clean. The day began with some dizziness. Was this something good happening to me, I wondered! Of course, everyone at home believed it was and with this wonderful thought, we rushed to the doctor. The result of the tests came in the evening. I was diagnosed with kidney disease. I understood nothing about it.

What did kidney disease mean and why did I get it?

Even as my mind was sorting out information, the change in the household's mood was so swift that I did not have the time to understand the disease or what it meant to my life and existence.

It became a daily routine. Sometimes as abuses and other times as bickering that continued through the day. I was trying hard to please them by playing a good wife and daughter-in-law while I was terribly confused about my health at all times. *Will I live? Will the disease take my life?* All the turmoil around, the verbal abuses, chiding me for things I didn't do or not accepting things that I did, kept my morale low.

My husband was an engineer; a professional. He heard all of this and never made an attempt to understand or correct his mother's perception. He never took time to sit and discuss or find out about my feelings.

I didn't know what to do. Cry about this marriage that was going nowhere or try to manage my disease?

After a few visits to the doctor and more tests, it was confirmed to be an autoimmune kidney disease. Some medicines were prescribed to manage my condition. The nephrologist warned me about pregnancy, saying it would be risky for both mother and child with my present condition.

There were days when I was barely able to walk to the toilet with the support of the wall. Sometimes I took the courage to call my parents and share my feelings which, when it came to my mother-in-law's notice, made her furious. Slowly, she spread the word among my other family members and friends in the city about my health and that her son was tricked into marrying a person with a kidney disease. Everyone seemed to believe that my parents had knowingly arranged my marriage.

At some point, she told me, "Your parents have not taken good care of you. They have neglected you, so your kidneys have failed."

My parents were heartbroken, not only because of the soured relationship, which turned into a torture, but they were also worried about my health. My mother mentioned it, reminding me of what had happened, "It's so sad that they were so keen on this marriage and they kept pursuing. Today, they forget that it was an offer from them and they were very keen on this marriage."

I would sit there feeling alone and abandoned, with no one to hold my hand and calm my nerves. Around me, there was no one who could show me love and sympathy. I continued to live in the house where there was no love for me. I had shared with my husband many personal matters, which he had conveyed to my mother-in-law, breaking the husband-wife confidentiality. So, gradually, I lost trust in the man I loved.

In those quiet moments, I would recall conversations with my parents. They would encourage us as kids saying, "Keep learning as knowledge is the best weapon that will come to your rescue" So I started courses to get more qualified, as a mere degree in Bachelor of Arts is very insignificant in today's world.

Suddenly, my mother-in-law sensed that money was being spent on my education, apart from medicines, so she started taunting me on a different subject.

"My son is already 28 years old, he needs a family with children," she would spell it out loud within my husband's hearing. So, even I had to consider this aspect as important. My parents were disturbed by this new expectation. They knew that the doctor had advised me against pregnancy, as my kidney disease would put my life at great risk.

I sat to think again, "A woman has to satisfy the husband and family in so many aspects. It is not important that I might not survive. As a woman, I'm a ragdoll to be verbally abused, to be treated with suspicion and left both physically and mentally shattered. To them, my disease means nothing. They divert my attention to other irrelevant gossip and make my understanding of the disease secondary to their needs."

I decided I would take the risk and give my husband a child.

In some time, I got pregnant. I continued to live in a hell where I managed the abuse meted out to me all through my pregnancy. It was a high-risk pregnancy and the toughest phase in my life, where I had multiple problems to resolve, with no shoulder to lean on.

I wanted to end my life several times. Suicide was constantly on my mind. But the little one in my womb made me want to live.

The child was born safely and that too within 3 years of my marriage. As much as I was emotionally exhausted with the marriage and the charade, there was no question of any separation from the marriage, as that was clearly not acceptable to my husband's family.

It was a few more years of maintaining my disease through medicines. Then, I needed dialysis or transplant. My father became my saviour. He donated me a kidney so that my life could get a semblance of normalcy. God has indeed blessed me with good parents and a wonderful 4-year-old.

What to hope for the future? I don't know, but I surely want to take control of my life.

Sheena Aurora

ADVOCATING BY PROFESSION, NOW ADVOCATE FOR AWARENESS

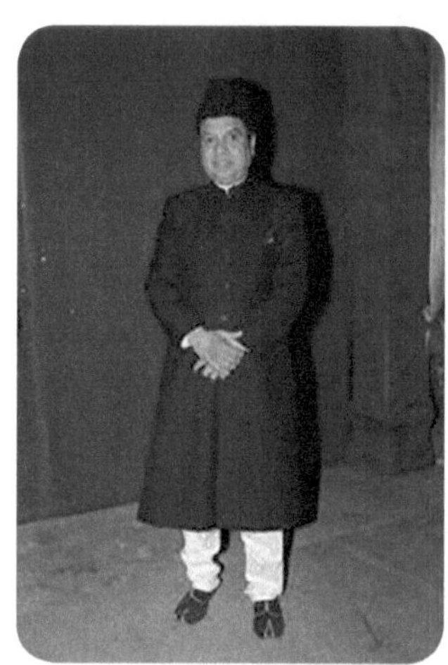

Hypertension

My back was wet with sweat. It was hot. I was thirsty. As I turned to lift myself up, my eyes felt the harsh glare of the sun. Opening my eyes, I realised it was the blue sky above and I lay in a bed of sand. My elbow brushed hard particles of sand.

"Just how did I reach this desert?" were my thoughts.

"Mariam!" I called out.

Gentle hands were shaking me. "What happened? Are you okay?" she said softly, as she always did.

Awakened by my wife, I sat up and narrated the incident. We both knew why my dreams were always bordering on loneliness.

This happened some 10 years ago when I was diagnosed with chronic kidney disease. As an advocate, I believed I was secure in all respects. I enjoyed a good clientele; enjoyed a good market reputation and the community saw in me streaks of leadership. On important matters, I was approached for my opinion. Financially stable and with family support on a strong footing, when the doctors mentioned kidney failure, I felt stranded as if I were in the middle of a desert.

I recall that day when my annual check-up was due and I was considering giving it a miss. When I discussed it with my wife, she said, "What's new? It's in your nature to think of all of us and our health, but when it comes to you, spending a few hours to get your health checked is difficult!"

I realised that I had upset her. To buy peace in the household, I went to the laboratory and got myself tested. It was 2 days later when my wife chided me, "So what about your blood test?"

"Oh, I forgot to collect my report," I said, a little annoyed for being forgetful.

When I collected the blood report, the friendly laboratory assistant spoke to me, "Please check your creatinine. Something seems wrong."

"What does that mean?" I asked casually.

"I think there's some problem with your kidney."

He added gently, "Go, see your doctor."

That evening, before going home, I met my doctor. We had a casual conversation. We talked about many things and the doctor enquired after my father's health. Then, indicating that I ought to lie down on the clinic bed, he began checking my blood pressure. As I looked at him, he simply said, "Your blood pressure is high."

He read the blood test report. "Creatinine is 2.8 mg/dl. I suggest we repeat the blood test. Sometimes there can be a mistake."

Taking his advice seriously, I got another test done the next day. It confirmed that my kidneys were failing. My family doctor recommended me to a well-known nephrologist.

The nephrologist studied my reports and ordered a biopsy. The cause of kidney failure was established. It was due to hypertension. Looking me in the eye, he said, "You can save your kidneys if you get strict with BP medicines and also follow a strict diet." He advised adopting a low salt diet with a small portion of good protein.

I settled with life with my kidney-friendly diet and medicines.

Sometime in January 2011, the blood test showed creatinine had spiked up to 8 mg/dl. When I met the nephrologist in 2010, my creatinine was still below 3 mg/dl. So, it always puzzled me. How could it change so fast? This was a situation I never dreamt about. I was very sad. I began feeling I should have stopped the creatinine when it was at 3 mg/dl. But honestly, my wife and I had worked well on the diet and been very careful not to miss medications. I knew the end of my kidneys was nearing. Very soon, I would need to start dialysis, my doctor had said. And then started all the series of dreams that put me in odd situations. Once I dreamt about being in the middle of the road with all the cars around me coming to hit me.

I decided it was time to talk to my family. In great detail, I discussed the matter, explaining my health condition, especially that I would be starting dialysis soon. Everyone was shocked and each one had something to say. Through all the chaos, few words registered, 'second opinion' and my mother saying, "*Darga manap.*"

Even before I could tell them to work hard to secure themselves financially, get independent and so on, all of them came forward to help me in every possible manner. I was so overwhelmed. Why did I imagine I would be alone! They were all clamouring to help me.

The best and most gratifying phone call was from my sister. "*Bhaisab*, I'm sad you didn't tell me about your kidney problem. I will donate my kidney." Her generous offer to donate a kidney to save me changed my sorrow to happiness. I saw all around me people who loved me so much and supported me so much.

The truth about most people is that until they are faced with a potentially grave problem, they never pause to think, wonder or organise aspects of life that's secure in their power. It needs a slight provocation, a hint of threat, to cause a ripple of fear down the spine or the stomach to churn for people to be moved to work towards bringing life's driving force under control.

A sudden change in the pattern of life, the edge of a cliff situation, triggers action in the right direction. Though financial security is always important, some frightening situations bring the realisation that it has been strengthened. When one faces such a threat, apart from finances, one needs a good network of family and friends to bring in comfort and solidarity. I realised that apart from getting a kidney donor, one needs to have good family support. I continue to be active at work and follow a daily exercise regime. Till now, *Alhamdulillah*, I feel good. I am truly thankful to Allah.

Apart from my personal health care, I have committed my time to spreading awareness about kidney disease. Early detection of the disease, monitoring blood pressure and diabetes and keeping vigil is most important. In the coming years, my group of kidney transplant recipients and I will conduct programmes to improve the lives of kidney patients.

Syed Mujahid Ali NaQvi
Transplant - 7 years

22 YEARS ON DIALYSIS – STRONG AND SMILING

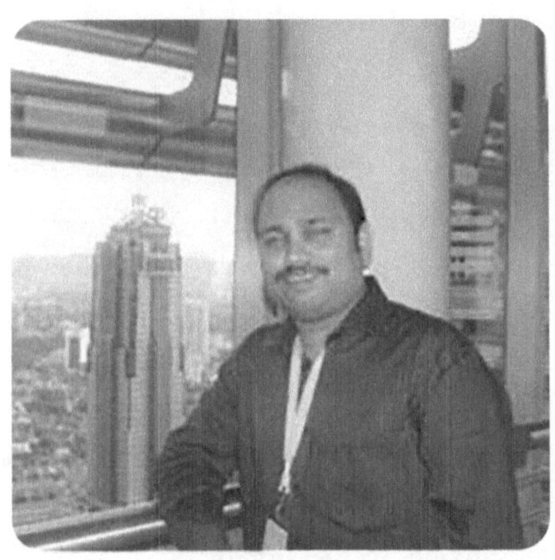

Neurogenic Bladder

It started as a breakfast conversation. Steaming hot *idlis* were served when Johnson spoke to me very excitedly about an idea that had struck him while driving to meet me. What he shared was the most wonderful concept. As I was eating, I listened casually at first and then with great interest. My friend talked about a revolutionary concept that will improve dialysis drastically.

He talked in great detail about how high-quality materials would improve existing dialysis. If supplied widely, it would mean good quality dialysis at the most economical rates. With the seeds sown, these thoughts continued to haunt me every day and so, doing my own search, I suddenly found myself getting excited.

This then became the concept of my business. Procuring high-quality material so that people at different levels of disease could get some customised dialysis. In my endeavour to improve my dialysis, I introduced high flux dialyser and many patients got an opportunity for better clearance of toxins.

I remember, my own understanding of the disease began at an early age. Diagnosed with chronic kidney disease at the age of 11, when most of my friends were still enjoying their games and schooling. I got my schooling as well, but additionally, was exposed to managing the disease.

The doctors said it was neurogenic bladder, a birth defect, which caused reflux, so urine went back into the kidney. This reverse process infected the kidney. Though very young, seeing my parents' expressions, I sensed it was a serious disease. Somehow, my parents didn't trouble me too much but always made me understand that I needed to take care.

By the time I turned 13, to improve the bladder's condition, 3 reconstruction surgeries were performed. But sadly, none of them really helped in improving the condition.

At 15 years of age, I had my 1st dialysis. Thereafter, a fistula surgery was done as a preventive measure. There was every indication that my kidneys would fail in the future, so the doctors advised me to maintain a protein-restricted diet.

My first reaction after I left the doctor was, "*Amma*, how does he think I can eat food that's without any taste? Even I want to eat good food like others!"

"If you eat as *Amma* prepares for you, it will be very tasty and good for your kidney. Don't you want to maintain it in this condition without dialysis?" *Appa* asked gently. "We want you to enjoy your life without going to the hospital for dialysis."

Though it was tough to miss out on good food, with determination I managed to maintain my condition, through my diet, for almost 10 years. I think full credit goes to *Appa* and *Amma*'s motivational talks and persistence in guiding me to easy ways to follow the medical directive.

Then finally, 10 years later, the day arrived. My levels had risen and I would need dialysis soon. However, as much I dreaded it, I had to prepare myself for this ordeal.

To my great surprise, the cadaver registration gave me an opportunity and a kidney was allotted to me. But within a short time, due to my primary health issues, the kidney was affected. It was tough to bid goodbye to my kidney. But my general attitude and my large group of friends helped me recover and accept dialysis as my best treatment. Initially, it was tough but in time I settled down with my new schedules.

Many years later, a friend asked me, "Ananth, are you the person who has been on dialysis for the longest time in India?"

I smiled, saying, "I don't know." But seriously, 1/2 my life was spent on dialysis.

I am now in the 22nd year of haemodialysis. During the process, one's understanding of the disease and how to manage it successfully are learnt through experience.

Today, my greatest joy is being able to eat everything and keep my levels under control. Without causing problems of excess potassium and phosphorous, by carefully choosing to eat in limited quantities, what modern nutritionists call 'balanced diet,'

I'm following it without even knowing I'm doing it. I also researched high flux tubings that improved my dialysis. This needed co-operation from the hospital and doctor. Understanding that for people on long-term dialysis this was important, they conceded to my request.

In April 2016, I became the founder and managing trustee of a trust, Kidney Patients Support Foundation. We lend assistance to economically backward kidney patients with medicines at subsidised rates.

In 2017, we branched out to conduct educational training programmes along with senior, experienced nephrologists to impart basic nephology in renal care to dialysis technicians. Advanced training is designed to handle all uncalled-for complications that arise during dialysis. Our program aims at reducing infection in dialysis patients.

My big dream is to have a caravan equipped with dialysis setup and travel across India to spread awareness of the disease.

In my 2 decades of dialysis, I have met many patients who grumble about dialysis, calling it unbearable. I think, since dialysis is the best option and many of us have little choice, we have to learn to accept dialysis as a way of life. Such an attitude will help people have a normal life. I enjoyed good support from childhood friends and my family, but nothing comes free. One needs to work to retain relationships. All this support has played a huge role and has helped me face all situations of life with courage and with a smile.

To me, joy also comes from outdoor activities, including long drives. It brings an appreciation of God's creations. One can just go for a walk to see his creations. An open mind is needed for everyone to admire the wonderful world we live in.

Ananth Pagadala
Dialysis - 22 years

CONCERN FOR AWARENESS IN SMALL TOWNS

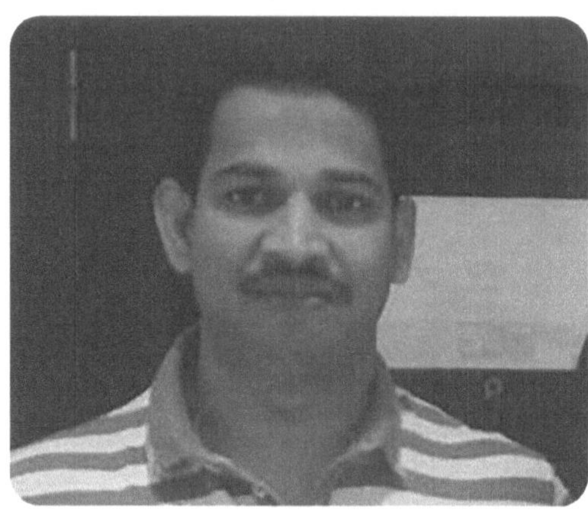

IgA Nephropathy

My eyes were almost transfixed. I vaguely remembered reading '2.0 mg/dl' and the biopsy report said, "IgA Nephropathy." What bothered me was that I am a doctor and that I should have known. I should not have missed the symptoms. How was it possible that I missed catching it early?

I thought about it for many days thereafter.

One day, I was busy with work when Nithya called. "Just wanted to check if you had lunch," Nithya asked. "I'm sorry. Will get it now," I replied, looking at the clock, which showed 3 pm.

"You're simply neglecting your health. It's always work, work and work," she got miffed and hung up with these words. Suddenly, it made sense. All the pieces somehow fit in. This was it, too pre-occupied. I never followed the rules that I made for my patients.

Years back, straight out of medical college, the passion to work for people who are in need of good medical services at reasonable rates made me decide to live in a town and set up practice there. I chose Kurinjipadi in Tamil Nadu's Cuddalore district. Nithya towed the line like a good wife. It was a small town but she adjusted to life there.

Our life in the small-town setting began early. Life was at a slow pace but for my wife, as a gynaecologist, and me, an ENT specialist, there was enough work every day.

People in the village were poor and they neglected many problems as it never struck them as important. When small problems are neglected, how fast it could escalate into a crisis. No human being gives it a thought in the course of everyday life. Their unique problem was always a challenge to handle, given their income levels, but they co-operated well in terms of following instructions.

Work generated through a network of general practitioners meant there was never a dull day in Kurinjipadi. My wife plays a great role in dealing with pregnancies and advising women on critical health issues.

Life was steady. The kids grew well, happy and relaxed in the simple village-like environment.

I read my blood test reports again. Yes, I must meet a nephrologist and get treated. What I advised my patients all the time was something I would have to follow now. Becoming medically compliant. What a new learning!

With the support of my family and good guidance from my nephrologist, I managed to stay away from dialysis for 4 years. It involved diet restriction and medications. The combination helped me achieve it.

When the dialysis began, it came with a whole bag of issues. For 6 months, it meant moving between the hometown and Chennai for the twice-a-week dialysis schedule. It was the most difficult period of my life, physically, to manage the rigours, the commute and attending to my patients. My health setback could not interrupt their medical treatment. They depended on me and as a doctor, I needed to show some responsibility.

But life had many more turns. The search for a donor began. Nithya was emotional when she blurted, "It's not easy to ask someone for a kidney." She knew well that only she could lead this part of the disease management. She talked to people in the family. It meant explaining how no harm would come to the donor, as during the testing period, the doctors would ascertain that the donor would be safe.

3 willing donors were rejected due to medical reasons. Finally, we found a distant relative who willingly came forward.

Recouping in the hospital after the kidney was happily settling down, I had some moments to think of other people. I had faced the harsh reality that anyone could have a kidney failure. In my case, it was due to abnormal deposits of protein. So, it was not that I was negligent or leading a wrong lifestyle. But will people from my hometown face such a situation? How many had the knowledge or the facility? How many could harness so much support? I wondered how many will have things falling into place finally.

Good that I had a health check-up so it was detected early. I thank God for this. My journey with the kidney disease has connected me with many people, some who have lived with dialysis for a very long time. One needs to understand the disease and decide to make some adjustments in life.

Dr. Raja Pooraswamy
Dialysis - some
Transplant - 2 years

JAPAN TO INDIA, WITH IGA

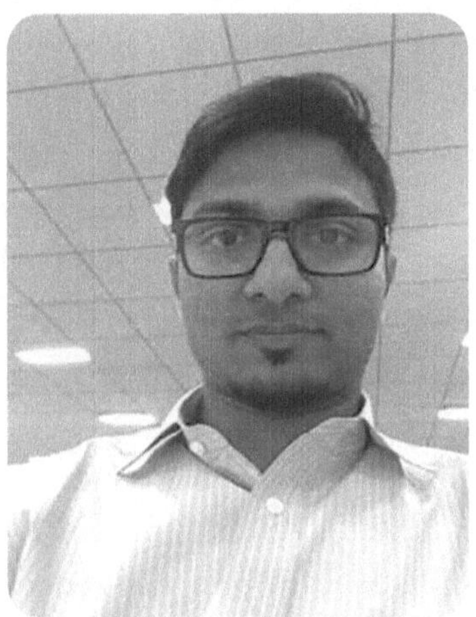

IgA Nephropathy

At 10 am on a Wednesday morning, the subway was not too crowded. As it came to a halt, I smiled at the lady with a kid and let them step out. Then, I hurried through a few blocks to get to Tokyo's St. Luke's International Hospital. As usual, I was a little concerned about the pain of the needle prick as I had an algophobia. I tried to calm myself.

At the pathology lab, I coaxed the nurse to be gentle with the needle. Samples were given for the annual check-up and I rushed back to the office for another long day's work. Life was just so good. I had a wonderful job, nice colleagues and a loving wife and kid.

Next day was a very busy day at work. I quite forgot all about the tests done the previous day, till I got a call from the medical care, asking me to go to the hospital immediately.

"Why are you asking me to go to the hospital?" I said without masking my irritation.

"Your creatinine is high. Please go to the hospital," she repeated patiently.

I was in a world where creatinine was not spoken about and I had never heard of it before. I kept arguing and she maintained the same reply. I fixed an appointment in one of the best hospitals. The doctor gently said he hoped the report results were false and that he would repeat the blood work to confirm it. He showed the result. The eGFR was 18%, so the doctor advised me to get admitted immediately.

I maintained that I had no symptoms and that I was completely fine. But he explained that further tests would confirm that my condition was serious. While returning home, I kept wondering, *How would I break this news at home without causing an uproar!* I casually told my wife what the doctor had said about my health. The next Monday, I got admitted for a biopsy of my kidney.

Every day, I underwent blood work to monitor my creatinine to check if it was rising. I was administered an IV of prednisone and had blood work almost twice a day. By now I had forgotten my fear of needles. The biopsy confirmed that I had IgA nephropathy. It was decision time; tough life and death decisions had to be taken.

I knew my family needed a larger family support and care during the emergency situation. I moved to Malaysia and kept a tab on my health with a good nephrologist. I was keen on avoiding dialysis and surgery by adopting a good diet. But the tables were difficult to turn. My health deteriorated and I felt continuous nausea, headache and physical weakness. At the same time, my work demands were mounting. It spiked my BP and my health began sliding down.

It was time to get a fistula fitted so that dialysis could be done anytime. I returned to India with urgency. With heavy nausea, I managed to get my fistula done in Chennai. My family members began offering their kidney.

Finally, I got a transplant. My mother gladly donated her kidney to save my life.

From a plush life in Tokyo, as a happy-go-lucky guy, I had to change my lifestyle overnight. My strong family support, their understanding and concern make me appreciate the extent of hardships people with kidney disease have to face. In Chennai's hospital corridors, I see real pain evident from the frown on their faces— it's financial constraints, hardships of life, travelling distances for treatment and so many other individual untold problems.

I wish to devote some time to work with a group of friends to alleviate the pain of less privileged people and help them find a way towards survival. I want to make every day count by the way I approach each day.

Kishore Kumar Palanichamy
Transplant - 2 years

MYSTERIOUS ENCOUNTER WITH CKD

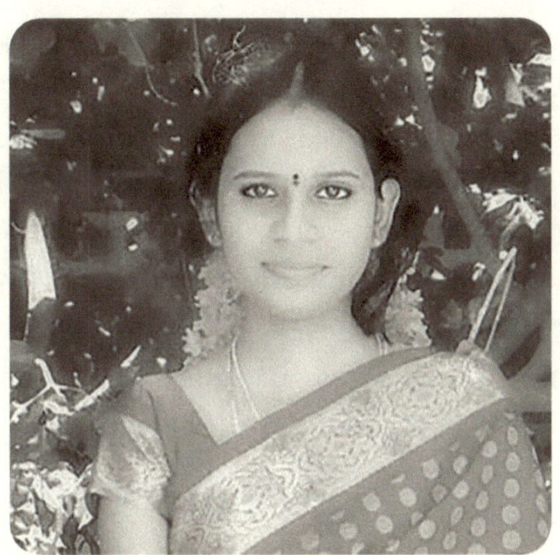

Drug Induced

I never expected my pregnancy to go so wrong. But at age 28, when I was due to deliver my 2nd child, it was an unimaginable horror not for me alone but also for my family who wondered if they would see me again.

It started when I went into labour. The pain had started and I got admitted to a small nursing home nearby. As expected, the family was totally excited, waiting in anticipation. "I think it will be a son. She has been so active during pregnancy," my mother had said, though she was worried and prayed that it'd be an easy delivery.

My husband was walking down the corridor as if his walking would make a difference. The nurses made sure no one entered the labour room. My daughter was dreaming about going home with a little sister or brother. So, there was a good build-up of excitement all around.

I was very confident about making it easy during the labour. The pain seemed so familiar and almost like the 1st childbirth. When did things change? I always wonder, even today.

At some point, there was excessive internal bleeding and I was wheeled in for a C-section.

This caused a wave of worry and the doctors asked my husband to sign a consent form as the operation was tricky. I was later told that there were plenty of alarming questions floating in the waiting room; some debate on "whys" followed by prayers, some agitation, so much so my husband had his hands full. He signed the consent form and things changed dramatically. It seems my son was in a tearing hurry and chose to arrive the normal way.

My darling son arrived, but I was in no position to see him! 4 hours after the delivery, my bleeding persisted. So, family members waiting in the lobby were panicking. "Why has the bleeding not stopped?" And speculative chats began.

Due to the heavy blood loss, I needed a blood transfusion. The nurses got busy hooking me to a stand for transfusion. But things went berserk. During the process of blood transfusion, I got infected. To save me, due to the critical condition, I was moved to the nearby Narayana Hrudayala Hospital. I was admitted into the ICU and placed under 24 hours of observation.

After 2 days in the ICU, the truth was out. I had a problem in my heart called cardiomyopathy, which is a heart muscle problem. Over and above that, my life was caught in the whirlpool of a life-changing disease.

The doctor declared, "You have CKD."

I asked, "So what will it do to me?"

He responded thoughtfully, "Your kidneys have failed. You will need dialysis to remove the toxins."

I was devastated. "Why has this happened? Was this due to some negligence?"

The doctor shook his head and said more to clarify, "Kidney failure can happen due to several reasons. Maybe you were given some strong medications and that affected your kidneys. But now, we will not be able to do any tests or biopsy to check what caused the failure of your organ."

I was moved to a ward and I struggled to fight my emotions.

It was so sudden and so shocking. The most tragic moment in my life! Even as I was struggling to find my peace, my husband became my greatest motivator. He explained how it was important to follow the doctor's advice and move on with our life. He brought the kids to see me. With the newborn in my arms, I became so emotional and burst into tears. But I saw the hard glint in my husband's eyes, of truth and support. Gradually, my fear melted into thin air and was replaced with a purpose to survive.

We discussed the options for dialysis with the doctor. I chose peritoneal dialysis, which I had to take 3 times a day. The hospital nurse trained me in the process of peritoneal dialysis and a dietician educated me on my diet. Peritoneal dialysis meant I had to learn how to manage it hygienically as there is a great chance of getting infected.

As I write about my experiences, I recall a conversation with a lady outside my nephrologist's clinic. She was in distress as she was to start dialysis soon.

I spoke to her gently, "Please don't worry too much. You will be fine."

"Are you also a kidney patient?" she asked, seeing my big smile.

"Yes, I'm on dialysis. As soon as you start dialysis, you will become comfortable."

Slowly, after some thought, she smiled back at me, holding back her emotions.

"You are very positive," she said.

This was what my family and friends had always remarked.

After spending nearly 2 years on dialysis, I managed to get a transplant. My mother was my saviour. Life is now as happy as can be.

The traumatic moments that day, when I delivered my son, seemed straight out of a movie. There was fear, worry and intense drama. I never knew what the outcome would be. My thoughts do travel back in time and I have to tell myself, "Move on, baby. There's a lot of work to do!"

Sandhya Vasanthakumar
Dialysis - 2 years
Transplant - 7 months

MANAGING TO STAY POSITIVE AFTER A REJECTION

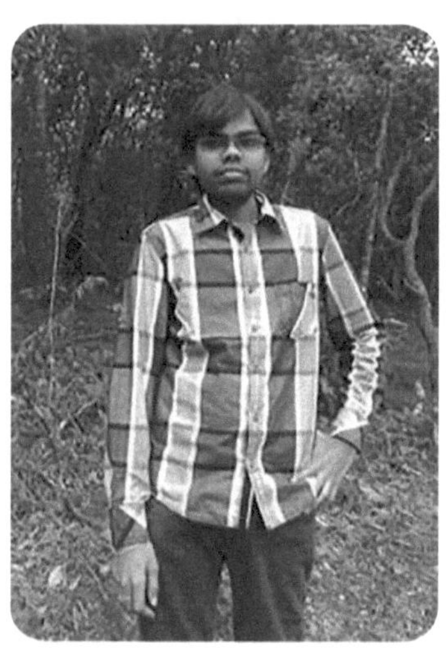

Paediatric Nephropathy

Have you ever enjoyed life in a village? My childhood was spent in Dalavoi, a village some 250 km from Chennai. My father worked in a factory and our life was fairly simple and peaceful. School was fun and relaxed, but I always wanted to finish school and go to the city for college. So, when I reached class 10, I got serious about my studies.

Our ordinary life suddenly turned into a busy one that needed us to travel from village to city to another state, all in search of solutions to problems. If people watched us do these trips in a hurried manner, without telling anyone, they would surely suspect us. But somehow, nothing mattered at that time as we were so engrossed in our worries. Our problems were all related to my health. Being so serious, it was difficult for us to talk about it to family or friends. During those trips by road and train, some of which were overnight travels, I grew up! I understood life had many things beyond our control and it was not child's play any longer.

If my friends were to call out, "Hey, Selvin! How are you?" I didn't know how to respond. I felt I could no longer laugh and talk to them about things we would freely do before. I felt like hiding away from them.

So, what had gone wrong?

One day, I had a stomach-ache, which in some time grew so severe that it would not go in spite of many home remedies. When the pain became impossible to manage, my parents rushed me to the hospital. The doctor who saw me was unable to identify what was causing the pain. He suggested that I be admitted to a local hospital.

After a week's stay in the hospital, when there was no change in the condition, the doctor suggested that we go to Nagercoil to Dr. Jeyasekhran Medical Trust. There were specialist doctors available there, who would be in a better position to help me.

This hospital had a urologist and luckily, a nephrologist consulted there once a week. By the time I reached the hospital, I was vomiting, not retaining any food, and there was swelling in my legs. So, when the nephrologist arrived, he immediately realised what my health condition was and declared in a serious voice, "It looks like Selvin has kidney failure. His blood pressure is very high, he is vomiting and there is swelling in various places." Touching my calf and ankle, he continued, "See how much water is here... Water stays in the body because he is not passing enough urine."

He spoke in simple terms, but my parents were speechless. This was the first time I had heard anything like that, so I didn't know what to say. In a complete daze, I began dialysis. Being in the hospital was a new experience. *Amma* was sitting there, crying all the time. It made me miserable, but I tried to hide my tears. Dialysis made me feel awful. I was wondering where and how I had landed there.

When we were going through so many issues, it was *Appa's* office management who understood the problems our family was facing. They knew this was a critical health issue and felt that I needed some good treatment. They provided many facilities so I could remain healthy. With their help, things were streamlined and I was able to travel in more comfort for dialysis.

Sometime after I started dialysis, I developed pancreatitis. So once again, it meant going to Cochin's Amritha Amma Hospital. A biopsy was done and they realised I needed further treatment. So, they started treatment with medicines for pancreatitis. I see this as the toughest time in my life. I had to finish my school finals and I had my dialysis schedules. Nothing made sense anymore. Somehow, I managed to finish my school exams.

When I sat by myself, I thought, "What options are there for me?" I needed a job, needed to earn and take care of myself. I could not sit and mourn.

But in some time, I began going to Apollo Hospital in Chennai to get better treatment. The nephrologist there assured me that I would be comfortable. After 7 months of dialysis at Apollo, I was feeling much better. At some point in time, we began planning for a transplant. My mother offered her kidney. In 2001, I had the transplant surgery.

Suddenly, life became so good and I was happy once more. I became the same old Selvin who was always jovial and enjoyed life. Now, I wanted to plan my future. So, I took up my education seriously and finished my high school. I registered for a Bachelor's degree in computer applications and things began to change. The kidney was slowing down and I could see my life falling apart. As the kidney gave up, it brought about a new problem. I got infected with hepatitis C. After a full course of treatment, my dialysis became my next pre-occupation. I was very sad with this setback.

Being so unhappy with dialysis, I began planning a 2nd transplant. But lady luck left my side very soon. I had a very high fever after the transplant and had to undergo a nephrectomy (removal of the kidney). So, it was goodbye to my transplant. I had to go back to the dialysis centre in Apollo Hospital thrice a week.

Throughout my time with CKD, I've been very aware of the importance of being employed in some productive work in order for my treatment to go on well. I learnt the importance of working hard to be self-reliant and becoming financially strong. But I feel the constraints placed by my dialysis, which doesn't permit me to perform better. Someday, in the future, I may be more successful with a transplant.

Selvin Raj Subbiah
1st Transplant in 2001-2004
Dialysis – 3 years
2nd Transplant -2007
Dialysis - 10 years now

SMALL SIGNS OF CKD

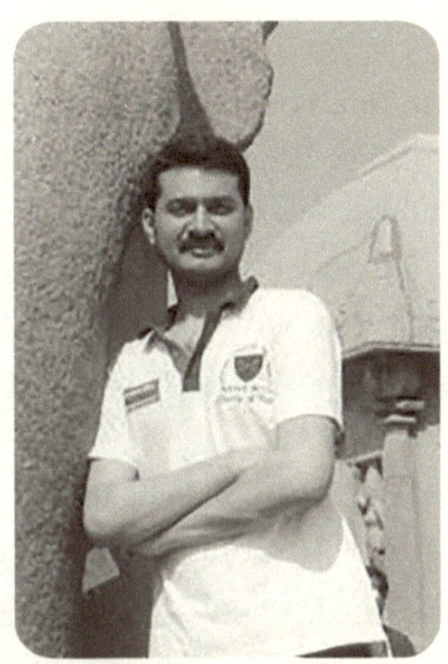

IgA Nephropathy

My story is a classic case of a young man growing up in a progressive-minded, middle-class family. I had working parents who were committed to the upkeep of their kids and instilled the importance of education. Love and respect reigned supreme in our household.

I spent all my life in Chennai. Life was good. I graduated as a software engineer and got employed in a reputed organisation. Life was brimming with opportunities—travelling overseas on projects and a large, good circle of friends. I was living my life to the fullest.

As I sit reflectively, I wonder, "Did I ignore any early signs? Was I too pre-occupied to notice them? Or was it sheer laziness as far better and exciting diversions stole my attention?"

This doubt bothered me and I started going back to those missed links, like when I woke up some mornings with a mild blur in my vision. I believed it would get resolved on its own and dismissed it, attributing it to sleepiness. On another occasion, I remember I had noticed a mild swelling and pain in my leg while going to bed. I believed I had resolved it by keeping my leg elevated by propping it with a pillow. I even experienced backaches but ignored them, assuming they were a result of wrong posture while riding my bike or sitting hunched while working on the computer. And at times, I felt I was over-sensitive to light.

Though I could say I was negligent and be harsh with myself, the clock cannot be turned back on what happened to me, how it turned my life and gave me life's greatest lesson.

I had seen job changes, shifted residences and in spite of the small murmurs on my health, I felt strong as if there was no force in the world that could stop my determined path to success.

What had been mere murmurs suddenly began sending strong signals. My body's temperature remained above normal and my weight increased dramatically. I would wake up with severe headaches, vomiting and the feeling of nausea remained with me throughout the day. When I scratched my legs, the itching was so insistent that the skin became raw; its colour and shine were gone. A certain degree of teeth discoloration was noticeable, gums bled while brushing, urine was frothy and my heart was pounding crazily.

One day, I gave into my eye blur and went to get it checked. The optometrist declared that my vision was fine. When I insisted my vision was not clear, the doctor asked me to do a blood test, an MRI scan of the brain and a digital retinal photography.

After the blood test and photography, I headed to another centre for the brain MRI. By now, I was anxious and fidgety. "Hope the MRI does not show something alarming," I thought, when the phone buzzed, as if in response to what I was thinking.

I answered my phone. It was from the eye hospital. The nurse spoke firmly, "Sir, please do not do the MRI. We got your test reports. So, stop the MRI and please come back here."

On entering his clinic, the ophthalmologist read the reports with a poker face and said, "The vision blur is due to hypertensive retinopathy." He checked my BP, which was 200/110 and then he revealed my other concerning parameters. They were way off the charts. The serum creatinine was at 9.2 mg/dl.

Then the doctor said, "The problem is with your kidneys!"

"You must meet a nephrologist soon. Please do not delay."

Though I realised it was very kind of him, my mind tried to reject his diagnosis. However, I could sense some panic building inside me. Getting proactive, I contacted a nephrologist and went to him with the report.

The highly specialised doctor was quick to confirm that, indeed, my kidney's function had gone to a dangerous level and that I would need immediate treatment. I felt as if I was sinking into a soft ground. Such devastating news was beyond my imagination. But prudence prevailed on me and I decided to take the next course of action seriously.

By way of further evaluation, a biopsy was advised. With great apprehension, I went through this invasive test, wondering what more would be known through this additional test.

The test confirmed my kidney's failing condition. The nephrologist explained that I had a rare disease called IgA nephropathy. The disease was lodging an antibody called immunoglobulin A (IgA) in my kidneys. This led to an inflammation that, over time, had hampered my kidneys' ability to filter waste from my blood.

Immediately, I was admitted to undergo a small surgery to create an access for dialysis. I was started on some BP medications and was ready to walk the journey of kidney disease. Before I got my bearings right, I was on dialysis. It took me a while to actually come to terms with my deteriorated health condition.

Throughout the tough period, I had support from family and my workplace. People understood, so keeping my cheer was totally up to me. In some time, I had begun looking at kidney transplant as an option; that would put me on steady ground and I could survive. But I needed to focus on getting the transplant right. I did a full study, found out information and started planning it properly. For that, the 1ˢᵗ thing I did was maintaining my health, with my levels of potassium and phosphorus within fairly normal levels. Sodium in my dialysis was restricted and I was regular with my medications. I wanted to be totally sure that I did everything, on my part, to make the transplant successful.

I had my transplant 4 years back and I am living life in the best possible manner.

CKD was just like a feather's touch. Thereafter, it is harsh reality, bringing a strong, life-long association with the disease. It's about management and knowing how to stay afloat.

"And then, there's no looking back," I said conclusively.

Senthil Raj
Dialysis: 1 year
Transplant in 2013

LUPUS IS DESTRUCTIVE

Autoimmune Disease

Banff National Park is God's ultimate creation, with the trees, shrubs and clear blue lakes. The reflection showed a woman smiling, but my eyes were shrouded in unspoken pain. I turned to look at my husband. He seemed relaxed, but I knew well how deeply he was affected.

I watched the distant hue in the sky and I started a page in my diary, inspired by the silence of the trees and lakes. I wrote slowly, thinking of the incident as it had occurred.

I was 33 years old, enjoying life and at peace with myself. Just as I believed, life was giving me everything, what with a loving and understanding husband and 2 marvellous boys. Suddenly, I saw my life take a different route. It was a severe pain in my finger joints that bothered me! Ouch! I never knew it was an important thing to notice. But that became the very 1st sign. Then, it grew to multiple joint pains, so I made my way to the doctor. I sat looking at the hard trunk of the tall coniferous trees, trying to collect my thoughts as I was still under the shock of the events that were clearly beyond my control.

At that time, my sons were 9 and 4 years old. Thoughts like, "What will happen to them?" troubled me. But their smiles and hugs tugged at my heartstrings and I knew I would fight tooth and nail.

So, I started some tests advised by the doctor. Seeing the reports, the doctor looked worried and said softly, "I suspect it to be lupus."

"Doctor, what does lupus mean?" I asked cautiously. This name was new to me, so I was now very alert, waiting to know more. But inside me, I could feel some uneasiness.

"It's an autoimmune disease. It causes inflammation like your joints have now. But let's get some more tests done," he concluded as if he wanted to avoid my questioning.

The test was called Lupus Antinuclear Antibody (ELISA). The test shows the presence of antigenic properties, primarily proteins, and detects hormones, bacterial antigens and antibodies.

My creatinine clearance tests showed things were normal. I was experiencing deep fear of the unknown disease. Why and how did I contract this disease called lupus?

The doctor said it could be drug-induced. But my other test results had shown lupus as positive. I was advised some medications for diseases of the connective tissue as systematic lupus erythematosus was one such condition. The drug came with a special warning, which the doctor had a good sense to alert me to.

I was not to step out in sunlight unless I wore full-sleeved, black clothes and carried an umbrella to protect me from the harsh rays. If the skin was exposed to direct sunlight, it could get discoloured.

To give the family a sense of moving ahead, a family summer holiday to Delhi was planned. I realised it would be difficult to wear the prescribed dress in Delhi's weather. So, I chose to skip my medications while on holiday. But skipping the medicines hit hard on me. My life was hanging with an uncertainty: how would this affect my health? It appeared lupus was around, rearing to grow huge. But no noticeable result was noted till after a few months.

It needed a test to find out my levels of creatinine had gone up, which was a sign of a kidney failure. Lupus had affected my kidneys, which I was warned against and which was my greatest fear. It seemed I had walked into the very dangerous zone. The biopsy showed I had lupus nephritis. I would need dialysis very soon.

It was a life of misery. I whined alone. In the hour of being low and extremely alone in the midst of a bubbling family around, I found much courage in Jesus Christ's altar, where I saw a bright light of hope. Over the years, I learnt to rely on the Lord during my weakest moments, finally seeing that the Lord was testing my patience. I realised that this was my life's chosen destination. Through some great providence, I received a transplant. It comforted me that I could avoid dialysis.

In a quieter moment, I reflected on my life and where I had reached. As if God sent me the thought, it appeared and I realised it. I had some severe abdominal pain due to my menstrual cycle. It was a tablet which was given to me without warning. This, apparently, could lead to a hormonal imbalance problem called drug-induced lupus.

Time has flown. My sons are now grown up, one even choosing his career. But I recall that tumultuous period of my life and as the disease raises its hood now and then like a snake, with minor problems, I feel it's still circling around me. It's not my imagination or apprehension. It is true.

I developed osteopenia, calcium deposits in the brain, symptoms of a tumour and varicose veins in my legs. Smaller issues such as dry eyes syndrome and losing teeth just like that trouble me, making me sound like a hypochondriac. If we sit and discuss our disease over a cup of tea, maybe that will reveal to us all possible dangers we are likely to experience.

In India, the awareness of CKD is low. Lupus has affected me so much that I was wondering how much everyone around would know about these severe diseases. Even today, I'm unsure of the extent to which lupus can harm a healthy body. In my experience, even some professionals are not really aware of the likely damage that lupus causes. Every day, I face some issues, small and big.

The problem is, people don't talk freely about health and more so, about serious diseases. These are kept as a big secret. Managing such a grave disease needs more information, such as personal experience and if it is shared, many people will be able to grow to understand the disease.

I have reconciled myself to the fact that my experiences with the disease will remain in the closet, behind closed doors, and freed when people walk up to me and ask, "How are you, Sudha?"

Sudha Kumar
Transplant - 12 years

HOW I LOST AN EARLY DETECTION!

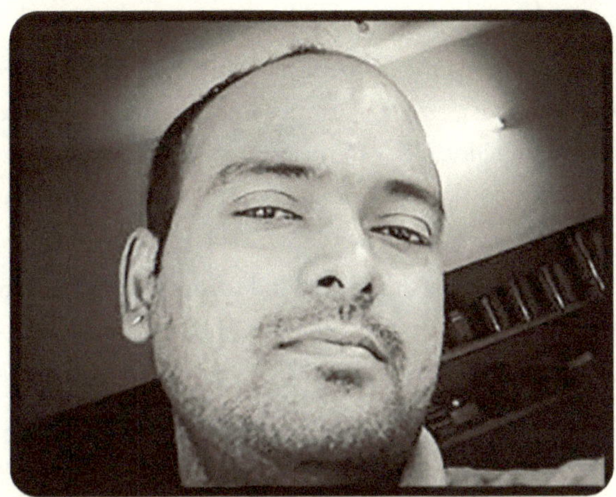

Hypertension

The doctor looked uncomfortable for a moment. It looked as if he was unsure, probably didn't know his job. I was told he was very experienced, so I had chosen to see him but now I was disappointed. "Not another one!" I thought to myself.

He simply asked, "Do you have a kidney problem?"

I glared at him and said, "No, only high blood pressure."

He looked at my swollen foot and said, "I'm suspecting it. Sorry, but let's do a blood test and see what the problem is."

The blood test confirmed the result. Yes, creatinine was very high.

The doctor said, "You need to get admitted to a hospital."

I nodded and left. I could not believe what he had said. My family felt there was some mistake, so we did another blood test and we saw the same result. This was the time of reckoning. I sat and thought of all that was wrong since November 2008.

It began with a headache. My physician confirmed it was due to high blood pressure and prescribed medicines to contain it. But my BP was very erratic. The doctor changed the medicines several times, assuring it would work in bringing my BP under control. No matter what, I continued to be in discomfort.

I had found it difficult to cope with office pressures. My uneasiness was growing each day, and slowly, the feeling of nausea became my constant companion. It had caused me great embarrassment one day when I vomited uncontrollably. Realising the seriousness of my health, my office granted me leave.

When my mother arrived, I finally had someone I could confide my miseries in. So, we met a new physician.

When he spoke, he clearly mentioned that when high BP is detected, a blood test is highly recommended. It was most alarming that the disease was left undetected. It meant I could have taken some steps to postpone dialysis. I was disturbed that the 1st physician had not identified the problem and alerted me. I lost a chance to take some proactive steps.

After meeting a nephrologist at the Apollo Hospital, I was admitted. As potassium was very high, emergency dialysis was needed. In the next 2 days, the biopsy result was out. It showed a rare kidney disease called FSGS and I was at CKD stage 5.

The treatment options of transplant and dialysis were discussed. To get ready for treatment, a fistula was created. Thrice a week dialysis began. Though my brother and mother were willing to donate, the nephrologist suggested that I wait for a cadaver donor. FSGS could affect the new kidney. So, I got myself listed in the cadaver registry.

When the going gets tough, many things go wrong. So, I lost my job. My close circle of friends extended rock-like support that helped me face the vulnerable period of uncertainty, emotionally as well as financially.

During my 5th year of dialysis, things changed. The hospital called, "We have found you a kidney."

My happiness knew no bounds. It finally worked. God has blessed me with a wonderful, working kidney, a supportive family and fantastic friends.

I will not forget my 17-year-old donor, Ajay, who gave my life a new meaning. I value his gift greatly.

As I reflect, I can vouch that no matter what, one needs to be informed about kidney disease. Firstly, if one has a high BP, get a blood test done. Secondly, if the doctor has failed to treat you after 2 rounds of treatment, get a 2nd opinion. Thirdly, stay away from all kinds of alternate therapy. One fools oneself thinking it will do the trick.

Lastly, and most importantly, always get registered for an organ transplant. If a family member donates a kidney, it is fine but the waiting period has to be

accounted for. There were a few calls and disappointments but finally, it happened. The first calls that didn't materialise were obviously for a good reason. They want to be sure the kidney is fit. Let's hope there will be a good conversion of cadavers into transplants so that many people struggling on dialysis have the hope to live longer and better lives.

Vinod Krishnan
Dialysis - 5 years
Transplant - 3 years

EMPLOYED, INDEPENDENT AND ON DIALYSIS

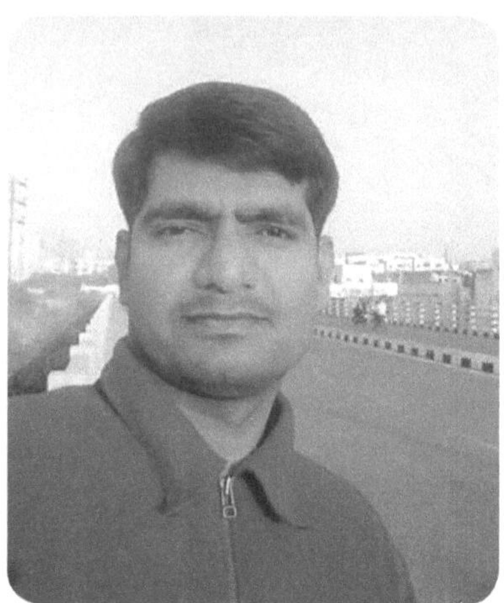

Hypertension

I always wondered why and how all this happened. How life had changed from happiness to this; lonely and disturbed. I was as normal as any young person, with some dreams for my life and future.

But things slowly changed. I was tired by the end of the day. Today, it was only working at the laboratory; tomorrow it will be a late night with dialysis on my schedule. That was the thing that bothered me when I was alone. When I sat with my family, they always tried to look normal. My younger brother would talk about his school and his friends and we would listen to him with a show of great attention.

Deep in my heart, I knew my parents were also sad. It was not easy to see such a drastic change come into our lives. Almost overnight, our happiness had shattered into pieces.

"*Appa*'s life has been such a long journey from the village to Hyderabad. I must always be careful not to cause *Appa* and *Amma* any more problems! After all, we are from a lower middle-class family." I frowned and reflected deeply on these thoughts.

I had such a great life just 6 months back. I had graduated in science. Our family income could not support further education. As the eldest, I realised my responsibility and looked for a job. With great pride and excitement, I took a job as a lab chemist in a growing industry. I would say the salary was good, meeting my expectations.

But that day in July 2005, our lives changed in a way that we had never imagined.

At some point, I noticed my feet were swollen. I visited a general practitioner, who checked my blood pressure, which was high. He advised a BP medicine to bring down my blood pressure. But a month later, my condition deteriorated and I was admitted to a hospital. After an ultrasound and a few blood tests, the verdict was out. I had chronic kidney disease and had reached the end-stage. Somehow, it made no sense to me.

I questioned, "Could things change in 1 month?"

"What does this mean? Kidney failure? Dialysis? How can this be?" my father asked, shocked about it. My mother was trying hard to hold back those big tears that were waiting to run down her cheeks.

I recall what the doctor had said, "Your kidneys have failed, get a transplant done as soon as possible." He said it in a professional manner but to my shocked ears, it seemed rude. (Today, as I look back, I understand why he had advised me!)

All of us at home knew that only dialysis was possible. Transplant? The thought of it caused great fear in us. Would we be able to handle it? It was such a huge step forward. Financially, it was far beyond our reach.

On 2nd August 2005, I had my 1st dialysis. It was a day of mourning for the whole family. No one knew what and why things were happening.

Through all the confusion around my life, I became aware of my company's Employees State Insurance Scheme (ESIS) that helped me get free dialysis. This was some sort of a silver lining to our 'grey, listless days'!

During the year, seeing me work so hard at work and undergoing my nightly dialysis schedules changed the mood in the family. They were willing to put in their last penny to save me. Both my parents tested for donating a kidney. My doctor declared that neither of them was a good match. For me, my brother was a kid. I loved him so much that I couldn't dream of taking his kidney. When it came to cadaver kidney transplant, it seemed very expensive to bear. So, I continued on dialysis.

Going to work during the day and dialysis at night 3 days a week cause more of a mental strain than a physical one.

Suddenly, the calm in the professional life was disturbed when the company was sold to a multi-national company and was shifting lock, stock and barrel to Uttarakhand. I was offered the position of a QA officer with a 5-figure salary. My dilemma was to choose between my health and good remuneration, which would also mean staying away from my family. With so much at stake on my health front, living with my family was a great comfort, so I decided to change my job.

It was most critical for me to join another company that was registered with the ESIS. I settled for a job in a small company as a data entry assistant with a 4-figure salary.

The question of whether I had made the right decision never crossed my mind! To me, the medical benefits through ESI that made dialysis free for me were the greatest boon. Today, as I reflect on my early days, I will vouch for the great management support during my tough times. They were always very accommodative. If I was unwell or late due to doctor visits/blood tests, they gave me concessions and were very considerate.

Meanwhile, I tried to maintain my health and fitness, going on early morning 5 km walks. I tried to remain as normal as possible with food, going out as other young men would, though I felt I lost much of my life's joys. Prayers and faith in God kept me busy and I tried to be a good person.

In 2012, I moved to a dialysis programme offered by Nizam's Institute of Medical Sciences, where I heard it was very good. I continued life on dialysis. This hospital was also covered by ESIC.

Very early on, I changed my food habits, eating simple, light meals that were suitable for renal patients. I was disciplined with both diet and dialysis. Though I was always tired, I would chat with fellow patients, sharing a few tips and knowledge I had gathered.

Another great thing that happened was, I got acquainted with Dr. Sree Bhushan in 2016. He spoke about the Jeevandan organisation that organised cadaver transplants. He encouraged me to go for cadaver transplant and I got myself registered.

My life changed overnight. A new hope, a yearning for a stable life, was something that could happen one day! Life through disease was good with support from family and friends.

Then finally, after almost 11 years and 8 months, I had a working kidney! On 22nd March, I got a cadaver kidney transplant. It was a very emotional moment for me. My family was overjoyed to see me happy again.

I learnt later that my donor was Satish. I thank him wholeheartedly very often, I'm also grateful to the Lord and to my family for their loving care all these years.

I sit and think of my life and understand what helped me all through the years:

- My discipline with dialysis and diet
- Faith in my family, doctors and following their advice

- Greatest decision I made was to maintain the ESIC status. Never letting any attraction deter me from my goal

- The 2nd best decision was to register for a transplant. I saw people avoiding taking the plunge

- I never took the route of breaking down, staying unemployed and becoming totally dependent on my father. Our humble background was always in my mind and I wished to remain grounded

Amar Nath
Dialysis - 11 years, 8 months
Transplant - 1 year

SOME CHANGE IN PLANS JUST HAPPEN

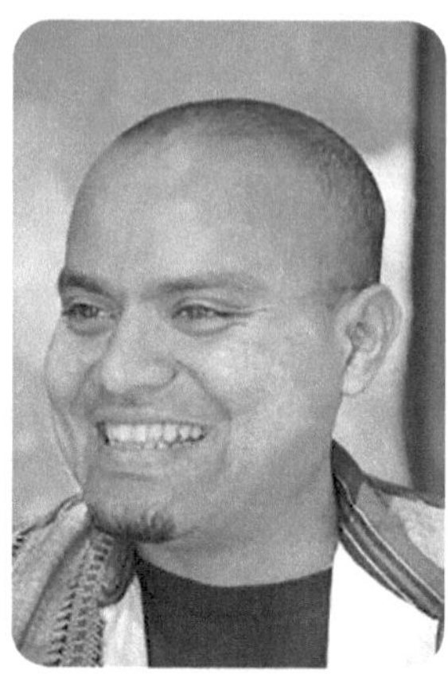

aHUS

I remember that day, 8th September 2007. I sat looking out of the window, seeing the trees turn bright after the morning dew drop. I turned and started punching my keyboard furiously.

"On July 14th, I completed 10 years with a kidney disease. What a journey it has been. The vaccines I took that day changed my life in a way I could never ever have imagined. What would life have been if the renal failure had not happened? I probably would have flown to the U.S. to join the University of Akron, armed with an I20 form (admission document), probably would have switched to MS (CS) in another university, would have completed it and then hunted for a job.

I would have worked for a few years and then would have gone to a business school and completed my MBA. Would have been working at another job. And yes, I would have probably even got married somewhere in between. A normal life, like most others.

How different my life is now."

When I read my blog now, almost 10 years later, with a smile, I wonder how I was so emotional at the start of the disease. Undoubtedly, I believe those major events shaped my next 10 years. A vaccination, a prerequisite for travelling to the U.S., showed me a new life. My being ill and staying in bed when I met the doctor who told me what was actually brewing inside me. The biopsy revealed a rare disease, atypical HUS that affects 2-3 per 10 lakhs (1 million) of the population.

As I stood feeling marooned, I did not see the irony of belonging to a privileged few in the 'rare disease category.'

Of course, I remember the failed transplant that happened after a few months of detection and how it destroyed me emotionally. It was the rise and the fall, so to speak. Then I had settled down to a life with peritoneal dialysis (CAPD).

Among the many things that I had always held close, being occupied with a job and entertaining myself were topmost. With these 2 requisites in place, it had been possible to live life to the fullest. My uncompromising attitude on these aspects made my life truly worthy.

Suddenly, thinking of the incident, I said to myself, "No, I can never forget that edge-of-the-cliff experience while holidaying in Mahabalipuram in 2004."

One moment, I was sitting and drinking tea, the next moment, I was lost in confusion. Suddenly, the sea's violent waves turned into the biggest tsunami seen by the world as it stormed in, destroying everyone who even remotely tried to control its wrath, and swept away many lives around me. I had no time to think and react while wading through the water-locked place that one can call debris. The next thing I had realised was that I had this series of horrific infections, ending with the much-feared peritonitis. It was a period when living was hell and death seemed like it was down the corridor. It had landed me in a great setback where CAPD was no longer possible. My life was a total mess. My doctor salvaged the situation by recommending daily nocturnal home haemodialysis. I was back on track with a life that I found meaningful.

Picking up my life, I started blogging, communicating the trauma of living on dialysis. I had co-founded a software company and during my spare time, I would do interesting things! I began blogging on any subject, including my health and life. Over 1,100 posts, 8 lakh views and almost 100 visitors per day brought me some recognition.

My many escapades with life-threatening circumstances include ventricular dysfunction and many issues with blood pressure. Oh, how I could go on. But none of it matters today. The early health landmarks will be my strongest link to life, other than my birth into a great family.

Vikram Vuppala, a seasoned healthcare strategy consultant with McKinsey & Company, U.S, began following my blogs on dialysis. Our casual discussions grew into a serious intent to change the way dialysis was done in India. So, my next great career opening came as a chance to be the co-founder of NephroPlus, which would eventually become the largest chain of dialysis centres across India.

In 2017, NephroPlus became India's largest network of dialysis providers. 126 centres, 81 cities, 16 states, 1 country. Many unconquered territories remain. The passion is still intact!

As a great advancement in thought process, NephroPlus initiated the Indian Dialysis Olympiad, making participants feel that there is life beyond dialysis.

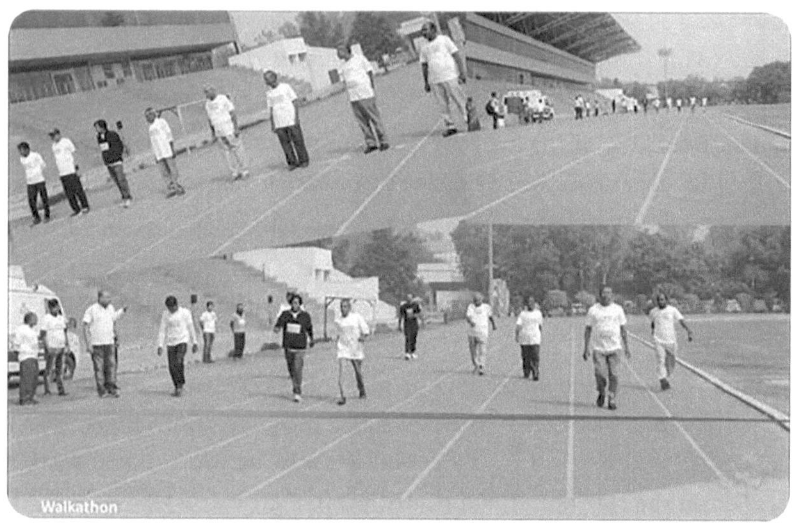

Handling kidney disease was one aspect of my life. I was now keen on creating more awareness about my disease. Very early on, I was told I had atypical haemolytic uremic syndrome (aHUS), a rare disease. But the true magnitude of the problem became obvious when many people, including doctors and other patients, looked surprised when I mentioned the disease. Most people hadn't even heard of aHUS.

So, I realised some awareness was needed. An in-depth study began to understand the future of people with aHUS and how they could get treated. My education as an engineer gave me a good understanding of CKD. A long-term dialysis person grows to become as good as a dialysis technician, understands the reports as if he's a pathologist, has broad knowledge about the disease, enough to discuss with nephrologists and to participate with other nephrologists in international forums and to organise research for kidney diseases.

Some factors that differentiate this disease are:

- aHUS is caused by genetic, chronic, very rare protein mutations that affect the body's immune system. The abnormality results in the chronic uncontrolled formation of small blood clots in the blood vessels all over the body.

- The disease affects adults and children. Recent imaging studies have enabled detection at the pre-natal stage.

- Though it is considered genetic, about 50% of the patients currently do not fall under any of the known mutation types.

- There's a chance of vital organs like the brain, heart and kidneys being damaged. Cases of premature death are also common. Many people need dialysis after they lose their kidney function. So, it is important to diagnose it accurately as early as possible. As aHUS has many of the signs and symptoms that are common to many other conditions, it is sometimes difficult to differentiate it from other conditions.

- Plasma exchange has been used, but as yet plasma therapy is not confirmed as the best treatment and may not be effective over a long-term period.

In the recent years, US' Food and Drug Administration (FDA) has approved Soliris (Eculizumab) for treatment of aHUS. Though there's great demand for saving many patients, the costs are very high for insurance companies and governments to afford it for the population they cover. This drug also has the potential to reduce antibodies in highly sensitised patients who are awaiting a transplant. So, with such varied applications, it would be great if market pressure could bring down its cost.

Today, I have completed nearly 20 years on dialysis. On a personal note, I'm active physically and enjoy a reasonably good social life with family and friends.

Though generally in a happy space, a few things still trouble me. I do hope a cure for aHUS would soon be available in India. After all, with such a large population here, even a rare disease will have a large number quietly struggling to survive.

The other major change I hope to see is the financial burden of the disease being shared by the states. How much can a common man pay? How many people can meet medical costs and manage to survive with a decent life for the rest of the family?

Kamal Shah
Dialysis - 21 years

PARENTS' UNDYING LOVE KEEPS ME GOING

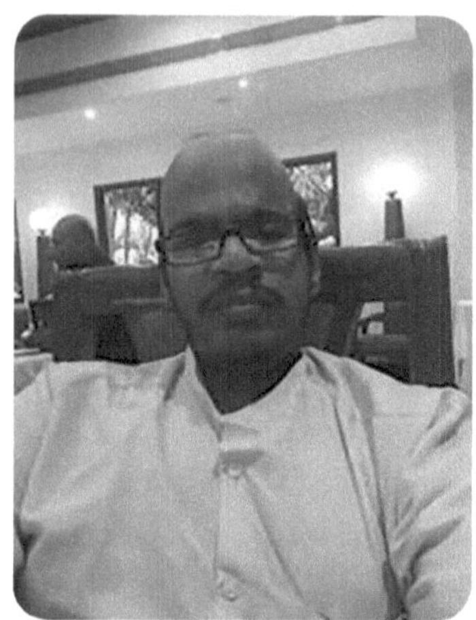

Spina Bifida

The husband and wife looked down at their pretty little newborn. They were in total disbelief that the little one could have any problem.

"He looks so normal! Why are they saying something is wrong?" she asked, with tears flowing down her cheeks.

Her husband gave a look of desperation. After all, he had no answer to such a fundamental question. His disappointment was not any less. Trying to console her, he summoned his courage and said, "Let us be a little patient. The doctors will tell us what to do."

It appears the few doctors who saw my case had a blank look on their faces. After much cajoling, my parents got to know more about my post-natal condition.

"Your son has what is known as spina bifida. It is a birth defect where there is an incomplete closing of the backbone and membranes around the spinal cord."

Shaking his head, he said, "Till now there's no cure for this condition. Chance of survival is very bleak."

I can imagine how much pain my parents would have faced, but they loved me deeply and they could never give up on me. Soon after birth, I was named Sai Krishna.

After checking with many doctors, my parents found a good experienced surgeon who could do a major surgery on me. It took nearly 6 months.

I want to say this, for a middle-class family in which both mother and father are teachers in schools in Khammam District in Telangana State, this is a very tough situation. In this district/town, hospital facilities are very limited. Even with the limited finances, they made extraordinary efforts to save me.

My parents had a huge stock of love in their hearts. They soon realised that the responsibility towards my future rested totally on their shoulders. After understanding the limitations that my health put on me, they began work right from scratch.

The 1st major hurdle was my inability to walk, which was directly related to my condition. Bed-wetting every other night was a routine that was accepted by them. All this meant a lot of physical work to handle on my hygiene and healthcare. Immobility, as I grew up, was overcome by using a wheelchair.

As both my parents were educated, they made sure my education was given top priority. They arranged for me to be taught at home, so I finished my schooling. When I was 15 years old, I visited a urologist. He advised me to start using a catheter. I felt better with this arrangement.

I finished school with good grades. From intermediate to my Bachelor of Technology degree, I attended a college. I remember how my father would drop me in college and pick me up in the evening.

It was almost like a gift to my parents when I graduated as a 1st class student.

I remember the day I graduated from college. My mother was so happy and she hugged me saying, "You made us proud, Sai." My father was also very happy.

Then things changed 1 day. I felt feverish and felt some heaviness as if I had gained weight. I woke up with a severe headache, vomiting and the feeling of nausea remained with me through the day.

The doctor advised some blood tests and a scan. The reports sealed my fate. My kidneys had failed and I was put on dialysis. This was in the year 2010.

With a desperate attempt to give me a normal life, my mother offered her kidney. But the doctor clarified that transplant was not an option for my condition.

Guess what? The latest romance in my life is with Hepatitis C Virus (HCV +ve).

While my journey with dialysis continues, I have fortunately met many friends who are long-term dialysis-dependent persons. They carry a torch that inspires me to live life.

What has life taught me? The many struggles that were part of my inheritance; struggles of my parents all these 30 years to see me live, breathe and enjoy life's beauty with a clear heart, clean mind and be untarnished by the bitterness of the wheelchair that sometimes cringes.

The memories of my life lie in the soulful music that keeps me company most often. It makes me see God and understand his overpowering role in my life.

Yes, I want to live. I want to work and be self-dependent.

Sai Krishna
Dialysis: 7 years

DISEASE MADE ME STRONGER

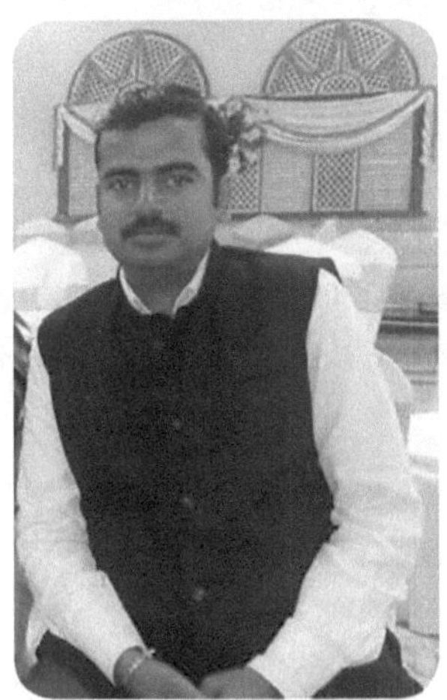

Hypertension

I recall a small incident in life, not long back. One that plays in my mind heavily so very often, as I question why I did not explore this further. It rings a bell of the most famous words, "If only…" These words are always running through our minds as we don't want to take responsibility for our inaction. But this becomes baseless when many things in life fall apart. Clocks cannot be reversed as per our command. It's totally our own mind that has to do all the questioning.

At some point, when I was 25, I visited a doctor. As is normal, the doctor checked my BP, gave me some medicines and as I was leaving, the doctor paused. Then he said, as an afterthought, "Just keep a watch on your blood pressure."

I didn't ask him why nor did he elaborate further.

Though it seemed irrelevant at my age, I decided to get a 2nd opinion. So, the next week, I visited another doctor. The 2nd doctor showed little importance to the question of high BP, waving it off. "You're young. There's nothing much to worry."

Relieved, I left the clinic after some small talk.

Why, oh why did the 2nd doctor waive it off? Why did I not go for a 3rd opinion? Again, no answer to such irrelevant questions that cannot be reasoned in isolation. Or did I go too fast and should I have waited for a few weeks to get an opinion?

Next year, I went for a check-up. My creatinine was 20 mg/dl and urea was 200 mg/dl. The doctor asked me to get admitted immediately and advised dialysis. How shocking! It was all too sudden!

I never understood then what these reports meant but had the good sense to start dialysis. Gradually, I learnt that my kidney's function was almost gone and it would have affected my heart if I had ignored the doctor. But the real understanding and acceptance took time to set in.

Life was now chaotic. **The dialysis and its routine made me very concerned about my future.** It had become complicated so early that I thought the destination, to reach any safety zone, was distant. **Though the doctor mentioned a transplant, I was not keen on disturbing my parents. There was a sense of guilt since I didn't take care and was most negligent.**

But I always noticed that family's support comes **at the best of times. It shows us how much one can love and gives us so much hope. I felt great.**

After a year, things started falling into place. My sister **offered to donate** and was tested. It was a perfect match and it was a perfect gift in every way. I got her kidney in December 2008. Our bond got strengthened and I'm living with all necessary precautions, enjoying life as before.

Through all this, I kept moving on in the professional front, adding many degrees. But my mind goes back to the period when my health was severely compromised but I was wonderfully rewarded with a 2nd chance at life. I feel a deep sense of gratitude for this opportunity.

Through the dark phase, it became clear to me that kidney failure can come in anyone's life. Instead of thinking that our world has come to an end, we must try to get back to a normal life. All that one needs is the support of family and friends.

But one thing I saw was, many people left me during the struggle; this too helped me as I could now depend on people who are real and solid supporters. The disease has given me new strength. My decisions are now more clear and strong.

Atul Pratap Singh
Dialysis: 16 months
Transplant: 9 years

IN STRIDE WITH CKD

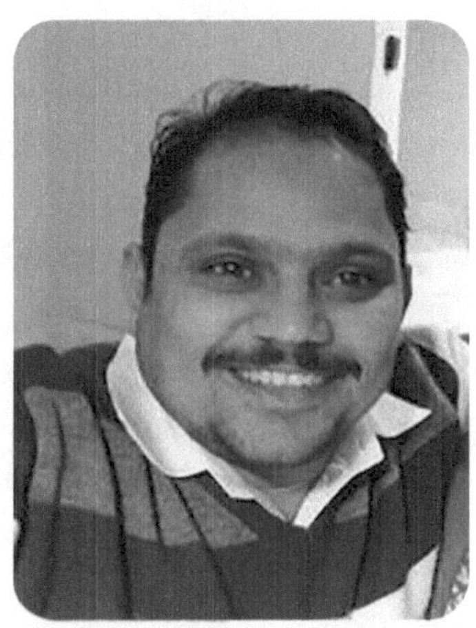

Neurogenic Bladder

My kidney story starts way back, at least 28 years ago, when I first met a doctor at Lucknow Medical College, barely understanding why I was there, at the young age of 4 years. Everything was new and enjoyable at that time. Few years down the line, after many more visits and continuous tests, I was told I have neurogenic bladder. What? I have been using this term for so long that it looks as if I understood these terms from the very beginning. But actually, over the years, with my practical experience, the terminology became clear. In short, it is the inability of the bladder to be emptied on its own.

What next? The same old story where parents try their best to ensure their child lives a healthy life, consulting one doctor after the other, from one hospital to another and even jumping from one specialisation of medicine to another. It is their deep desire to solve the problem for their child. Over the next 24 years, they did everything sanely possible to ensure a remedy. They tried Allopathy, Ayurveda, Homeopathy, Yoga, other alternative medicines and so on.

In between all this, I was continuously trying to live a normal life as I never believed something was wrong with me. Though my parents did all the exploratory work, they let me believe that all was in fact well with me. From a very small age, the doctors told my parents that their child would have to use intermittent catheterisation whenever I had to answer nature's call. I know this is too technical, but I used a catheter, which is a plastic tube, every time I felt the need to pass urine. So, I do the same activity 3-4 times a day; every time, till date. Think about how tough it would have been for a school kid to do that in school.

Over the years, this continued and along with that, all the experiments to ensure I get well soon continued happening. Over the years, blood tests which were conducted every quarter started revealing problems with kidneys, so by the age of around 9-10 years, I was told my kidneys will get damaged sometime in the near future. From that day onwards, the caretaking routine of managing my kidneys started leaving all the tasty food out of my diet to ensure my kidneys worked longer. No tips were known on what I could eat and what I couldn't. But the only thing I remember is, 80% of all meals were *moong dal khichdi.*

This diet management and other restrictions allowed me to live normally for almost 24 years without moving on to the next step, which is renal failure. Finally, the doctors suggested dialysis for which I needed lots of mental preparation. This was really next to impossible. Now, after being on dialysis for the past 10 years, I think others should take hope from my challenges.

The question everybody asks me is, "Why don't you go for a kidney transplant?" Let's remember the beginning, having neurogenic bladder means a cure needs to be found for the bladder first. If that's not corrected, a transplant would not be possible. Many doctors have confirmed it would be the wrong decision to go for a kidney transplant.

I go for dialysis thrice a week, a schedule that I have followed for 10 years. So many life-changing experiences happened, some were life-threatening and changed my entire outlook on life. One thing I loved about being put on dialysis, all food restrictions were mostly gone and water restrictions came in. So, after a long time, I was partly happy as I could eat different things apart from *khichdi* and a part of me was not happy as dialysis is not the most enjoyable thing in life.

Why did this happen to me? People are with CKD because of high blood pressure, diabetes, stress, accidents on road, taking wrong pills and so on… So, this is something I wonder about often!

I have not even revealed the most interesting part yet. At birth, I was diagnosed with meningocele (again, too technical), a swelling caused by protrusion of the covering of the spinal cord. I needed a serious operation. Imagine the pressure on the doctor to find veins in a 2-day old baby, in absence of facilities like MRI and CT scans! By the grace of God, the only side effect happened to my bladder and the rest is history, which I shared with you already.

But all this as a part of life was totally worth it. I am happy doing things with friends. I constantly make changes in the way I live. Life is only because of that.

I LIVE MORE AND ENJOY MORE!

Mohit Dhawan
Dialysis: 10 years

WHERE DO I START?

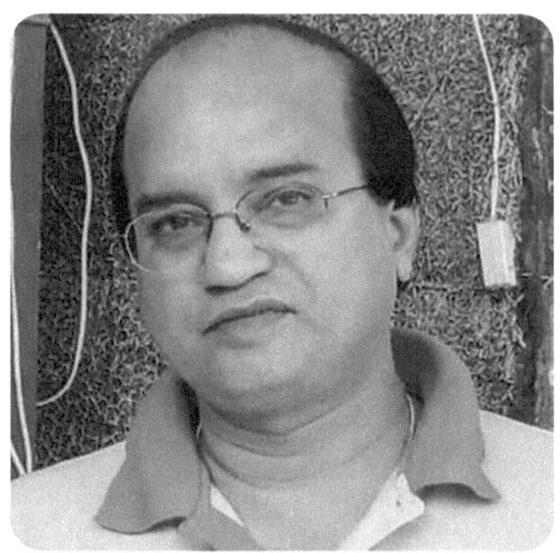

Diabetes

I saw myself at the edge of the cliff in 2013.

It had been tough to manage my health. My son got married but while the arrangements were being made, I had to manage my health with some treatments. After the marriage, things went out of control and I had to be admitted to Lucknow's SPGI hospital. I was vomiting and had severe abdominal pain.

It was finally detected as chronic kidney disease. After the initial shock, I disclosed to the doctor, "My health history began in January 1996 with diabetes. I thought everything was well. No one mentioned anything about 'creatinine,' ever! Even the 2013's report had shown creatinine at 2.35 mg/dl and now, in 2014, it is at 3.00 mg/dl or in that range!"

I saw the doctor nodding and smiling sympathetically. But what could he do?

As I returned home, I was thinking deeply, "Is this now my end? Am I really dying?" Even when my mind started calculating my days left on planet earth, I realised I had unfinished duties. My daughter had to be married. I immediately diverted my mind to prayer instead, worshipping fervently.

My daughter got married in 2014. I'm grateful to God for making it possible.

My next deadline: September 2017- March 2019. I need to be in perfect condition during this period. I want to work and retire with my good health. I'm keeping my diabetes under strict control. Sometimes the creatinine creeps up, but I started walking regularly and do yoga, apart from being regular with medication and diet.

Diabetes is a dangerous disease that quietly ruins our health. Everyone must check their health at regular intervals. Diabetes is not age-related. It can occur at any age.

Shivkumar Tiwari
Varanasi

ALPORT SYNDROME AFFECTS MORE THAN KIDNEYS

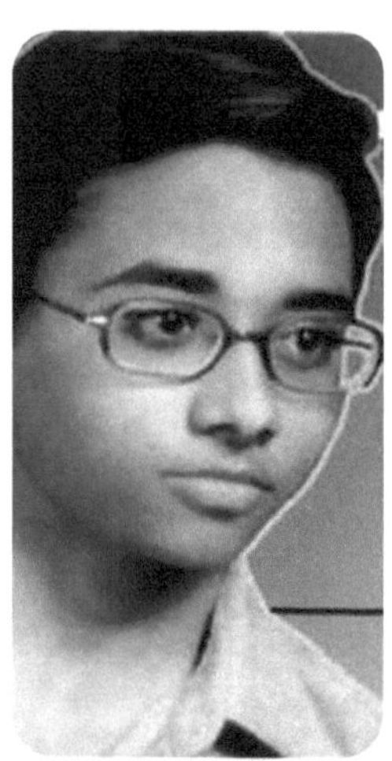

Alport Syndrome

No one knows what will happen the very next moment in life. One just lives life as each day unfolds. I was a carefree person, a 20-year-old in college, doing my intermediate college.

Dehradun is the best city. All my childhood was spent in this city of dreams; the hilly terrains and the green beckoning landscape made it ideal for my dreamy state of mind. I had cherished my share of dreams of a future that had lots of fun and music. It had travel, it had some career plans and my heart swelled with hope and happiness.

Suddenly, my heart missed a beat. *What's happening to my eyes? Why is my vision blurred?* My mirror showed some injury in my eyes. In the next 3 months, this condition occurred thrice. I was in great agony and was worried too. A visit to an eye specialist gave us the first surprise. He said it was not an eye problem, but he sent me down another road, to meet a nephrologist.

Meeting the nephrologist led to many tests that revealed a serious condition. Looking at me with concern, the doctor said, "Your blood test shows creatinine above the normal range. It's high at 4mg/dl." A biopsy confirmed that it was Alport syndrome, a genetic disorder. The doctor spoke gently in great detail and explained the treatment.

Apart from some diet restriction, I had to take medications to maintain my kidney condition. The doctor had hinted at dialysis and transplant as options. All those valley dreams came tumbling down because not only did the threat of the dreaded 'dialysis' loom large, but many issues of my blurred vision disturbed me. I lost the zest to go back to complete my education, with many health issues cropping up now and then.

Somehow, with family support, I managed to deter dialysis for 8 years. In that period, I lost so much weight that after 2 attempts to create a fistula for haemodialysis, dialysis was done using a catheter. Then, we decided to do peritoneal dialysis thrice a day. My movement out of the house got further restricted. To be useful to both myself and my family, I engaged myself in home-based professional work.

How has the disease impacted my life? Issues with BP led to swelling in my face several times. Weight is currently 39-40 kgs. The struggle due to low weight is a major issue that I encounter.

But more than that, to me, my family's life bothers me. The medical expense is huge and my family is burdened by the recurring medical expense. My father's income at the court is insufficient to manage my treatment costs. Some part is managed through assistance from CM Relief Fund, some friends, relatives and NGOs. But how long can we manage like this?

When a disease comes into a middle-class family, apart from the patient, everyone suffers. It is emotional. It is financial. It is also hopelessness. It is the loss of quality of life.

We muster all our courage and try to face the world, without being limited by disease, but a happy future is evading us.

Mayank Singhal
Dialysis - 2 years, 8 months

LIFE WAS BEYOND ORDINARY

Alport Syndrome

When a child is born, parents rejoice! They have the world's most valued possession. They begin to check the newborn; are the legs, arms, fingers, toes and all other features fine? They want to know if everything is working perfectly. As the child grows, they wonder if he can speak and then they marvel at his 1st word. All they can think of is to shower as much love and care as they can. This is their true wealth.

I was one such child. My life was total bliss. For a long, long time I believed I had everything in the right compartment. If you thought of a family, I was born in 1978 to young, lovely couple. I may have cried because of a fall or an ache, but never because I was naughty or because my parents were angry with me. I was a happy child and the world was a wonderful place to live in. Being a good, obedient and caring boy, things worked wonders for me.

I performed well at school. I was that kind-hearted person who helped people. Total strangers regarded me with respect and trust. Lifting spirits of the poor was something I simply did because of my own sense of compassion. My parents were always proud of me as I was a conscious student with the right attitude.

My childhood story could have been a fairy tale where we lived happily with no worry. I'm happy but I feel shy to say this, I fell deeply in love with an amazing girl in my high school years. She was so unique and it was such an instant liking. It was as if my life depended on her.

But to do anything, I had to secure my life.

For further education, I chose engineering, passed the entrance test and joined a prestigious engineering college. I gradually lost touch with the woman I loved. I was sad that I never had the courage to tell her what I felt for her. But very soon, a tornado rocked my life.

I was sick, very sick, and was detected with Alport syndrome. I had no idea how such a horrendous disease entered my life. We were simple people who only knew simple living with high values. Our philosophy of loving and sharing had no place for medical emergencies. But solidarity was the topmost family strength. Exploiting our strength, my mother took courage and got me treated at Vellore hospital by donating her kidney.

With determination, I finished my studies, became a civil engineer and began working at a government job, where I worked for 10 years.

This was a happy period for me. I suddenly wanted to trace my friend, the lady I loved. Finally, when I tracked her down, I found out that she was married and had children. I was shattered that life had given me another blow. But gradually, I consoled myself saying marriage is difficult for a person who is post-kidney transplant. People need security.

Now, 17 years later, my kidney has again failed. I'm back on dialysis and hating it. My parents are old and very hurt that my kidney failed again. They suffer from disappointment, just like I do, and ask God why I am being punished.

With Alport syndrome, life is complicated. It impairs sight and hearing, so one feels lost in this loud and noisy world. The dialysis, the kidney failure and the trauma of the syndrome's impact on the faculties combine to make life very difficult.

The next stage of dialysis with no hope for a 2nd transplant makes me sad. How will life be? How can I continue to make my parents proud?

Sumanta Dutta

CKD IS FOR BOTH RICH AND POOR

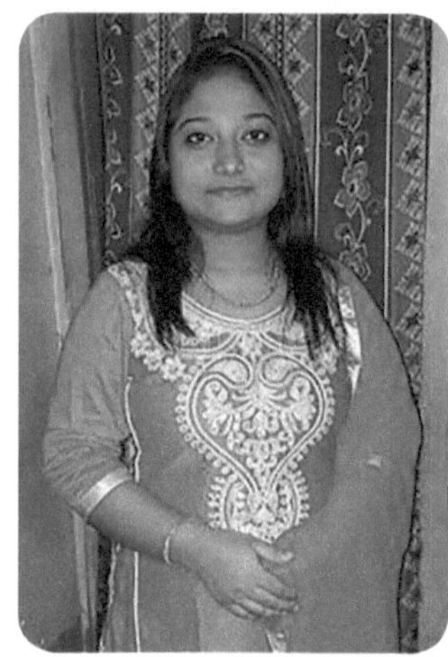

Hypertension

I stood looking at the doctor. I totally rejected his diagnosis. Just because I was vomiting for 5-6 months, it did not mean I ate things that cannot be digested.

He had said, "You have a kidney failure."

My mind was thinking fast, "What's he talking? I'm not a rich person, eating richly prepared food and consuming alcoholic drinks or eating cakes!"

"But doctor, there's some mistake. I eat simple, home-cooked food. How can my kidneys fail?"

The doctor explained, "You are not the first person to say that. Every one whose kidney fails thinks it is some fault with their food habits. Kidney failure happens due to many reasons."

Later, when I sat by myself, I remembered all the patients I had met in Kolkata and all the hospitals in Delhi. After all, I had seen as many as 7-8 doctors in the past few months.

In those hospitals, I had seen many types of patients: some very rich, counting diamonds on their ring; some from the middle-class, worried about their medical bills and others who were poor, simply waiting. So yes, kidney disease is every man's disease.

I was an intellectual, book-loving person. I was a gymnast and so, physically active too. What hurt me was, I was in Delhi looking for a job after my post-graduation and my health was now in a mess.

As my doctor read the report, "Creatinine is 5 mg/dl," I got tense. My cousin, who was with me, asked a few questions, "Doctor, what is the treatment? Will medicines help?"

"Dialysis and if a donor is available, you can have a transplant," he said, looking at me kindly.

I had met a doctor in my hometown, Kolkata, where in response to my vomiting episodes, a kidney function test was conducted. Creatinine was high and so was the level of urea. When he suggested a transplant, we had to shy away as it was expensive. So, I knew my chance of survival was bleak.

I knew how difficult it was for my family to manage the day-to-day needs. Getting a job in Delhi would have been of great help. After knowing this background, I was not thinking of troubling my family. How will my family raise the 4-5 lakhs or more that will be needed for a transplant? I was very upset and worried that life getting so complicated.

But sometimes, there's an extraordinary power that makes it possible! It happened that way for me. Through some clever planning, we managed to raise partial funds. Seeing our plight, my cousin gathered forces and managed to help us.

When good luck shines, all good things happen. My mother felt encouraged with all the efforts around fund collection and she happily stepped forward to donate her kidney to me.

The kidney transplant surgery went off well. Now, I'm maintaining my health and doing everything possible to keep myself healthy.

Kidney failure is not only about the disease. It is about managing to find funds for survival. Many people like us find it very difficult. But if one tries and plans well, people around come to our rescue. In my case, I was very lucky that my mother was healthy and could donate. So many aspects come together to make way for a kidney transplant.

Also, just as disease can come to rich and poor, people who are poor can also survive. One has to work towards it. God always blesses us for our efforts. We must never lose hope.

Swaralipi Nandy
Dialysis: some dialysis
Transplant: 4 years & 8 months completed

PART – 2

Our purpose behind adding some pertinent information on medical aspects of the disease is to offer guidance to patients and provide information that will give some perspective on issues around the disease. Some senior nephrologists have been invited to help us in this section. For more in-depth information, you may read journals and other medical books.

This Section Deals With

- *Prevention of chronic kidney disease*
- *Living kidney donation is a gift of life*
- *Overcoming challenges of donor adequacy*
- *Kidney disease: where is it heading?*
- *Emerging rock star: IgA nephropathy*
- *Understanding dialysis and its value*
- *Guide to read your lab report*
- *Patient-centric aspects: trauma and need for support*
- *Facebook chatroom*
- *Facing a kidney failure*
- *Glossary of technical terms*

Thank you.

PREVENTION OF CHRONIC KIDNEY DISEASE (CKD)

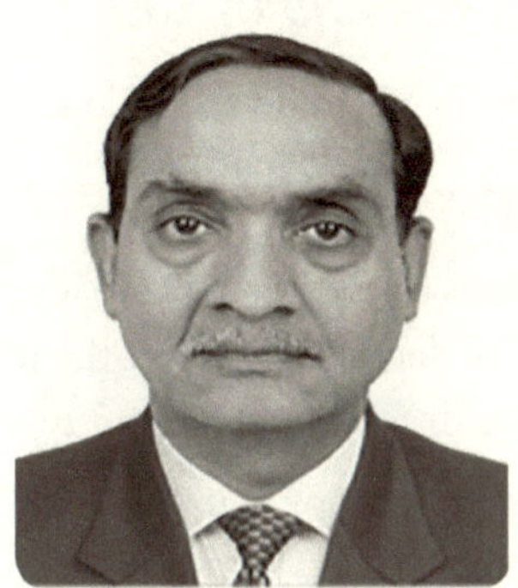

Dr. Sanjay K. Agarwal

Kidneys diseases are of 2 types: acute kidney injury (AKI) and chronic kidney disease. AKI develops from a few days to weeks, and most often, it is curable. However, CKD cannot be cured.

The definition of CKD for a layperson:

- Kidney damage as confirmed by
  - ✓ Urine analysis showing abnormal findings (high protein and abnormal cells)
  - ✓ X-Ray and other radiology tests of kidney showing abnormalities
- In some people, there could be significant decrease in kidney function
- The condition persists for more than 3 months

Unfortunately, once CKD is correctly diagnosed, the patient cannot become normal and the disease is likely to progress to reach end-stage kidney disease (ESKD). CKD will worsen with time from stage-1 to stage-V. At end-stage kidney disease, stage-V, nearly 90% of kidney function has been lost. The time to reach ESKD may vary from patient to patient. Once the patient reaches ESKD, the options for treatment are either life-long dialysis or a kidney transplant. At this stage, medicines alone will not be able to maintain the life of the patient.

How Common Is Ckd in India?

CKD is currently a serious public health problem all over the world, including India. It is estimated that approximately 3–4% of adult population in India has some form of CKD. If you see 100 healthy looking people anywhere in India, at least 3–4 of them will have some degree of kidney disease.

Investigations and Diagnosis of Ckd

For the diagnosis of CKD, one needs to do the following tests:

1. Tests for Diagnosis of Kidney Disease

1st step is to be certain that this is a case of CKD. To identify it as kidney disease, some tests are normally required. The doctors will select the tests needed for each person, as conditions may be different for different people and types of kidney disease.

- Simple urine examination for protein, sugar and cells
- Blood creatinine and urea
- Plain X-ray kidney, ureter and bladder area
- Ultrasound abdomen for kidney, ureter and bladder area

2. Tests for Diagnosis of Chronicity of Kidney Disease

For the diagnosis of CKD, we need to confirm that kidney disease has been persisting for more than 3 months. There are not many tests which can show if the disease is chronic kidney disease. It is often a clinical diagnosis by observing tests over a few months if they are available. Otherwise, urine examination, ultrasound and sometimes kidney biopsy are useful in making this assessment. Best way to understand chronicity is to compare tests over the last few months. Therefore, it is important to maintain a record of all the medical tests done in the past.

3. Tests for Diagnosis of Cause of Ckd

After concluding that it is CKD, we need to do other tests to find out the cause of CKD, as it will help in better management of health. There are many causes for CKD, so doctors will obviously need clear information to decide the course of treatment. Some important tests for detecting the cause of CKD are:

- Urine examination
- 24-hour urine examination
- Plain X-ray - kidney, ureter and bladder area

- Ultrasound for kidney, ureter and bladder area
- Blood sugar
- Eye examination
- Other tests

CKD is a life-long disease, progressive in nature and incurable. We should try to prevent CKD from reaching end-stage ESKD, at which phase the treatment options are not easy for a common man.

Prevention of CKD

It is a well-known fact that in early stages of CKD, many people do not have any symptoms, making early diagnosis and prevention a little difficult. We need to specifically look for CKD by investigations. One option is to look for CKD in the whole of India. But in view of the very large population in India, this approach is not possible. Another approach is to look for CKD in specific groups of patients where chances of CKD are high and in fact, this approach is also being followed in many countries like USA, UK, and many others.

Following High-Risk Groups of Patients Need Screening for CKD

1. Patients with diabetes mellitus
2. Patients with hypertension
3. Patients with family history of diabetes, hypertension or kidney disease
4. Patients who have symptoms suggestive of kidney disease

1. Patients with Diabetes Mellitus

30-35% of patients with diabetes mellitus will develop CKD at some time. Across the world, this is the most common cause of CKD. Therefore, patients with diabetes mellitus need regular screening for CKD. In patients who have insulin dependent diabetes mellitus (IDDM), also called type-I diabetes, urine examination for microalbumin should be done after 5 years of diagnosis of diabetes. If microalbumin is present, then appropriate action needs to be taken. If it is absent, the test may be done at an interval of 1 year. If the diabetes is Type-2 or Non-Insulin Dependent Diabetes (NIDDM), then urine test must be done at the time of diagnosis of diabetes and then it should be on the person's annual medical test list. In addition to urine examination, the patient must do all other tests that are advised for the management of diabetes.

2. Patients with Hypertension

10-20% of patients with hypertension may develop CKD at some point in time. It is more common if blood pressure remains uncontrolled. It is highly recommended that persons with hypertension should have adequate control of their blood pressure. Also, they should get urine examination for protein done annually and if urine protein is found, appropriate action needs to be taken to manage it.

3. Patients with Family History of Diabetes, Hypertension or Kidney Disease

If any member of the family has diabetes mellitus, hypertension or CKD, other members of the family are at a risk of developing diabetes, hypertension and CKD. So, first-degree relatives of this person also come under the high-risk group for CKD and should also be screened for not only diabetes and hypertension but also for CKD.

4. Patients Who Have Symptoms Suggestive of Kidney Disease

In addition to the above 3 groups, patients with certain symptoms should definitely be screened for CKD. These symptoms include:

- Swelling of body
- Unexplained weakness for many months
- Unexplained low haemoglobin
- Bone pain and bone fracture with minimal trauma
- Person having recurrent infections, including urinary tract infection
- Loss of appetite and tendency to vomit for a long period

What Action Is Required Once Ckd Is Diagnosed on Screening?

Once the screening diagnoses CKD, the following action is needed to revert kidney damage or decrease progression of CKD to further stages:

1. Weight reduction, if patient is obese
2. Less salt and sugar in diet
3. Limited fat in diet
4. Strict blood sugar control, if diabetes is present
5. Strict blood pressure control, if hypertension is present
6. Stop smoking

7.   No regular painkiller and no painkiller which has 2 drugs in the same tablet

8.   No medicine on their own

9.   Medicines to decrease protein leak in urine like angiotensin-converting-enzyme inhibitors (ACE-I) and/or Angiotensin Receptor Blocker (ARB)

Dr. Sanjay K. Agarwal
Professor and Head
Department of Nephrology
AIIMS
New Delhi-29, INDIA

LIVING KIDNEY DONATION IS A GIFT OF LIFE

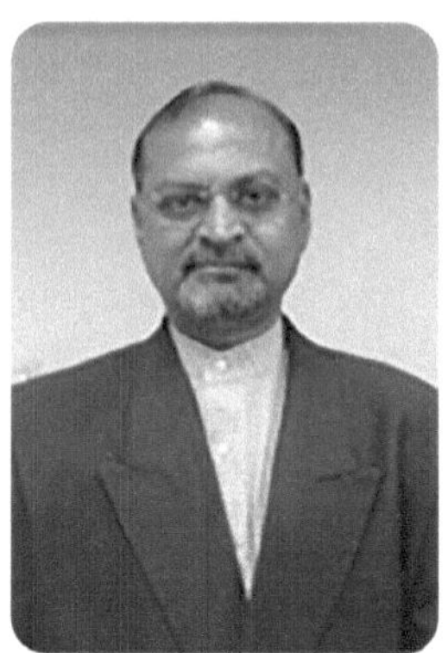

Dr. Sundar Sankaran

When I chose nephrology as my specialisation, the attraction was to work in a complex, emerging field where so much mystery was being unravelled. Gradually, city-by-city kidney transplants, as well as dialysis as a survival treatment, grew in prominence, and I'm glad it's across the length and breadth of India. Affordability among Indian patients is a growing concern for patients and nephrologists as well.

Years back, I would return home unhappy when one of my patients couldn't survive. Today, in the 21st century, we are struggling to understand numbers of kidney transplants conducted, people who got into dialysis and people who couldn't manage to continue their brave fight.

The complexity of the disease has grown multifold, even as new solutions to mysteries are announced each day.

Over the past 3 decades, in my personal experience and as also as per practice established world over, the best way to treat ESRD is with a kidney transplant. Kidney Transplantation done with a Living Donor is easy, with cadaver donor (also called Brain Dead Heart Beating Deceased Donor), it needs a registration process and for Unrelated Living Donor, the rules are long and cumbersome for the aspiring donor to willingly comply.

According to the Indian law, any living person can donate, if medically fit, to a close relative (definition of a close relative - parents, siblings, spouse, children, grandparents). All others are considered 'Unrelated' or 'Non-Relative.'

Unrelated donor transplants need to be cleared by the Government Authorisation Committee. The process for unrelated is tough and each state interprets the law differently.

The differentiation between procedures for related and unrelated donor transplantation acts as a deterrent for people choosing a kidney transplant. The Government Authorisation Committee has the role of determining if the unrelated donor is a willing donor who is not coerced or that there has been no financial exchange involved. While this is a good safeguard, in execution it becomes a very lengthy process, delaying genuine cases. Such watertight laws also create a fear of legal action. This acts as a deterrent to living donors who offer to assist with a kidney donation. Delays at various levels have led to increase in mortality.

The supply of kidneys through the cadaver programmes is low in India as compared to western countries. Some corrective measures to make more patient-friendly laws must be reviewed on a war footing. All my years of work have been to save people who face extinction due to a kidney problem that accidentally came into their lives. This need to review laws is expressed only to save many patients from succumbing to the disease. Please know that I'm not advocating organ sale or exploitation of the poor.

Kerala's model, introduced by Father David Chiramel, where unrelated donors became Good Samaritans by donating a kidney under his Trust, Kidney Federation of India, has served many patients well. The priest donated a kidney to a poor man, thereby leading this altruistic movement.

If every state in India can have an NGO doing similar work, many people will see happier times and lives will be saved.

n attempt to motivate kidney patients to find their survival path is the vision we need to hold out to them. It needs fuller support and understanding, by the Government, of the trauma and challenges that affect patients when trying to fight for survival.

Dr. Sundar Sankaran
Consultant Nephrologist
Head- International Transplant Services, Manipal Hospital. Bengaluru
Chairman, Indian Society of Nephrology (South Chapter).

Overview of India's Kidney Scene

Guesstimates of kidney patients, transplants and dialysis

	Guesstimates	
Incidence of ESRD	250,000	250 per 10 lakh population
Transplants in a year	5,000	10% cadaver
Dialysis	100,000	80% leave treatment
Patients added each year	250,000	70-80% start dialysis

*Source Dr. Vivekanand Jha

OVERCOMING CHALLENGES OF DONOR ADEQUACY

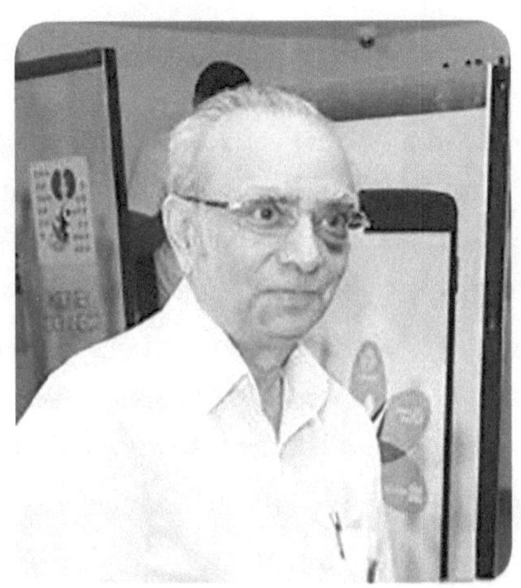

Dr. Bhupendra Gandhi

Historically, one has seen how researchers and sharp thinking minds have found routes to rescue many lives through their struggle with chronic kidney disease. After many trials in 1954, the 1st kidney transplant with twins made it easy in the absence of anti-rejection medication. Even as early as 1955, research for different blood group transplants was conducted, only to conclude it would not work. Today, we call it *ABO Incompatible kidney transplant. *ABO incompatible transplants attempt to increase donor pool and overcome the blood type barrier using the desensitisation protocols.

When nephrologists see many patients succumb to disease, fresh thinking and outlook have come to their rescue. Constant innovative methods have emerged through developmental work by researchers and sharp thinking minds.

Few great measures that are now widely used:

1.   ABO incompatible (ABOi) transplants

2.   SWAP or Paired transplants

After the first attempt of ABO incompatible transplant in 1955, by incorporating the desensitisation protocol, the concept was explored in 1987 by Alexandre et al, making way for successful ABOi transplants. Japan used this technique widely in 1989, over

1000 transplants were conducted as deceased donor transplants were almost negligent. US and Europe followed through later in 2000.

India too is now equipped to conduct ABOi transplants. In 1989, the first of such transplants were handled under my supervision. Thereafter, in Mumbai, over 100 such transplants have been conducted with good success rates. Now it is gaining momentum and many large centres in India have been successfully implementing it.

Recently, India had to its credit the first ABOi transplant in kids in SAARC countries, conducted at Medanta Hospital.

The SWAP or Paired kidney transplants also had its genesis many years back in 1986, when the concept was shared by Rappaport but only in 1991, it was attempted by Dr. Park in South Korea. He and his team were leaders who used this unique approach to increase transplants to beat incompatible donor-recipient issues.

Later, in Switzerland (1999), in US (2000) and many countries slowly established themselves. Though this is a novel concept, it faces implementation issues causing extraordinary wait time. The exercise is time intensive and involves lots of advocacy.

India has made a fair in-road into SWAP. Much more coordinated effort will bring better results.

For better surgical efficiency and accuracy, robotic transplants are being done in several cities in India. It will add to graft survival with minimum complications in surgery.

There is serious intent to review and improve laws, such as considering adding many more relationships to be accepted as legitimate for organ donation.

In years to come, the artificial kidney that's under advanced clinical trial stage in the US is likely to reduce many woes for kidney patients in India as well.

Dr. Bhupendra Gandhi
Consultant Nephrologist, Jaslok Hospital and
Research Center and Breach Candy Hospital
Mumbai

KIDNEY DISEASE: WHERE IS IT HEADING?

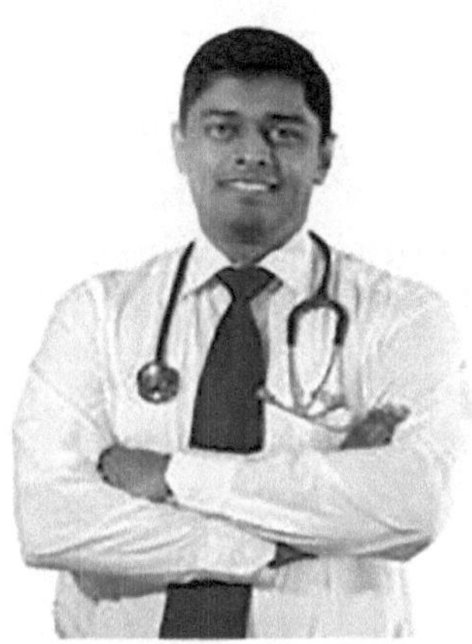

Dr. Avinash Ignatius

Some Estimates and the Global Burden of Disease Study's Predictions

CKD has resulted in almost 1 million deaths worldwide and 1 out of 57 fatal outcomes is a direct result of CKD. It is 1 of the few growing causes of death. CKD was the 13th leading cause of death in 2013; this compared to 1990 when it ranked 27th, a rise of 134%.

A study published in American Journal of Kidney Diseases projects that the number of new cases of chronic kidney disease (pre-dialysis) will grow significantly through 2030. More than half of the U.S. adults aged between 30 and 64 years are likely to develop CKD. The prevalence of CKD in adults 30 years or older is expected to increase from 13.2% currently to 14.4% in 2020 and 16.7% in 2030.

Over 2 million people worldwide currently receive treatment with dialysis or a kidney transplant to stay alive, yet this number possibly represents only 10% of people who actually need treatment to live. More than 80% of all patients who receive treatment for kidney failure are in affluent countries with universal access to healthcare and large elderly populations. In middle-income countries, treatment with dialysis or kidney transplantation creates a huge financial burden for the majority of the people who need it. In another 112 countries, many people cannot afford treatment at all, resulting in the death of over 1 million people annually from untreated kidney failure.

Kidney disease is closely inter-related with heart and blood vessel disease, with 1 out of 16 of all cardiovascular deaths being attributed to the reduced glomerular filtration rate (GFR), a principal marker of CKD.

CKD also has a strong impact on quality of life. According to the Global Burden of Disease, Injuries and Risk Factors (GBD) study, among over 300 causes accounted for in the study, CKD is the 15th leading cause of years lived with disability and 20th leading cause for disability-adjusted life years.

Many of the large epidemiological studies conducted in different parts of the world reveal that 10–13% of the adult population have markers of CKD. Kidney diseases are projected to grow further due to many factors, including the ageing general population and the growing prevalence of diabetes.

Although the prevalence of CKD is common, and it has a high impact on mortality and morbidity; directly through kidney diseases and indirectly by increasing cardiovascular diseases, it is not recognised enough as a public health issue.

Non-communicable diseases (such as diabetes, heart disease or kidney disease) have replaced communicable diseases as the most common causes of premature death worldwide. An estimated 80% of this burden occurs in low or middle-income countries and 25% is in people younger than 60 years.

Chronic kidney disease can be treated. With early diagnosis and treatment, it's possible to slow or stop the progression of kidney disease. Modern clinical practice guidelines for CKD are available and the appropriate treatment has been developed for protecting kidneys. Implementing the available cost-effective treatment has already helped to delay CKD complications in distinct subgroups of patients in the emerging world.

However, in many countries, the medical personnel responsible for managing acute and chronic kidney diseases is scarce. Patients don't get detected or screened early or are not referred to a nephrologist early enough. Therefore, evaluating and treating kidney disease should be a part of the medical curriculum and postgraduate training of all clinicians, regardless of their subspecialty.

Kidney disease is common and harmful, yet treatable. To combat this growing challenge and achieve better health and economic sustainability, kidney disease should become a part of national health plans along with strategies to increase public awareness.

Dr. Avinash Ignatius
MD, DM,
Senior Consultant Nephrologist,
Pune

EMERGING ROCK STAR: IGA NEPHROPATHY

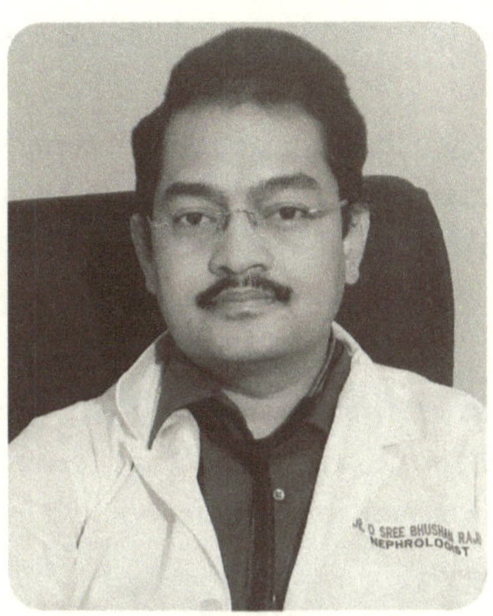

Dr. Sree Bhushan Raju

In recent years, kidney disease is on the rise. Research has shown that apart from hypertension and diabetes, significant growth is coming through rising incidence of IgA nephropathy.

Though IgA nephropathy ultimately leads to kidney failure, there are some interesting aspects that keep it different from other kinds of kidney diseases.

Background: IgA is an antibody that protects the intestinal tract against bacteria or other viral infections. This antibody is found in the mucosal covering.

over the intestine. Some genetic aberration changes the character of IgA antibodies, which begins sticking together in the blood, forming large molecules. Glomerulus, which plays the role of the kidney's filter, has small pores, making filtrations of large molecules impossible. Unfiltered molecules get deposited over the glomeruli, damaging them. This results in proteinuria, a protein leak through urine. Abnormal protein entry into the urine tubules gradually reaches the kidney tissue, creating further damage.

An interesting aspect of the IgA is that many people don't experience symptoms like other kidney diseases. The disease takes the route of a slow developing IgA or an aggressive kind that quickly leads to kidney failure.

The absence of "kidney-disease-like symptoms" does not rule out some other indications. Some people find blood in the urine, which is known as macro haematuria.

Blood is sometimes invisible until noticed under laboratory urine tests when micro haematuria can be detected. These come as stray incidents and hence can be missed. It will be preceded by some viral infection involving the throat, which will clear after a few days. Such patients will face very less proteinuria and the blood pressure could also be normal.

One can safely say no treatment is needed and even kidney failure may develop after a long time.

Managing the progression through control of hypertension is particularly helpful, so the rise of creatinine is gradual over several years. But if at detection, the patient has swelling all over the body, one may find a major protein leak of around 3-4 gm/ day. If this condition does not respond to treatment, the kidneys could deteriorate over the next few years.

Cases of people with severe hypertension and rapid rise in creatinine, which shows as a crescent in the kidney tissue, will manifest in a severe and rapid variety of IgA nephropathy. There is little response to treatments and it escalates into kidney failure, requiring dialysis or transplant.

Associated Complications

- Hypertension damages kidneys and puts a strain on the heart and blood circulation. High blood pressure should be treated vigorously.

- If IgA develops slowly, one must be aware of any sudden change that comes into notice. Research has shown that in 20% of cases with slow progression of ESRD, it would take almost 20 years to reach the end-stage of kidney disease. But it isn't the same for all cases.

- There may be protein leakage from the kidneys. This may be slight and only detectable in urine tests or occasionally, there are high levels of protein leakage, leading to swollen ankles and high levels of cholesterol in the blood. This is called nephrotic syndrome and requires specialist assessment and treatment.

- IgA nephropathy has a variant called 'Henoch-Schonlein purpura.' In this, the IgA antibodies affect not only the kidneys but also other parts of the body. A blotchy red rash may appear on the legs and buttocks. However, if one has had IgA nephropathy confined to the kidneys for some time, chances of it converting to the more serious Henoch-Schonlein purpura have not been recorded yet.

This is not an easy condition to treat and usually, doctors rely on treatment of hypertension, control of cholesterol and managing changes that take place due to kidney damage, like in other cases.

There is some evidence of some patients with deteriorating kidney function being helped with steroid (prednisolone) tablets. But complications due to steroids are expected and this does not improve health for all patients. Some other drugs have shown improvement in few clinical studies. Fish oils administered earlier are now no longer prescribed, as results were not encouraging.

Future of IgA

This disease is fairly new. Research is being conducted to understand the spurt in the spread of IgA in South East Asia, including China, India and others. In most cases, this condition does not affect normal life. It does not require any special diet. One continues to be physically active. IgA has not shown signs of inheritance, so that makes it far easier to handle. However, for planning a pregnancy, a patient should discuss with a doctor and take precautions needed for pregnant women with kidney problems.

There's a possibility of IgA nephropathy returning to the new kidney after transplantation. But there is little chance for another kidney failure.

Dr. Sree Bhushan Raju
Professor & Head
Dept of Nephrology,
Nizam's Institute of Medical Sciences,
Hyderabd, Telangana

UNDERSTANDING DIALYSIS AND ITS VALUE

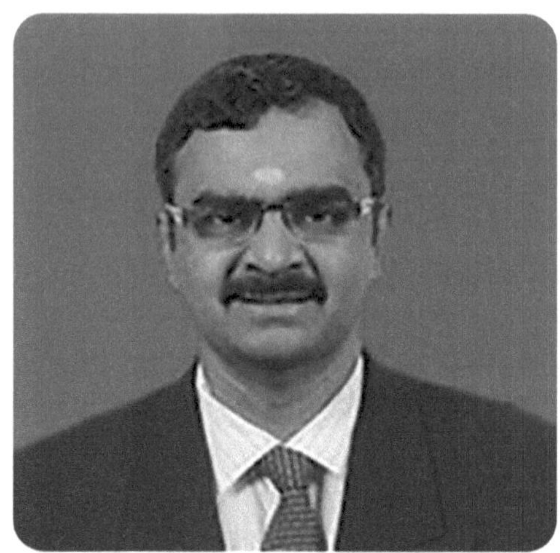

Dr. Raju Balasubramaniyam

Dialysis is most often the first stage of treatment as kidney transplant is a time-bound process. When patients are detected with chronic kidney disease in advanced stages with high levels of creatinine and blood urea nitrogen, dialysis is the best and speedy treatment to remove the build-up of toxins. AV fistulas are created for dialysis at the wrist to connect an artery and vein through which the blood purification takes place. Fistula generally needs to be planned in advance as it takes time to mature and become functional. These are safer and more hygienic from the point of infections.

The biggest challenge faced by the patient and the family is to understand the disease and consequences of delay in starting treatment.

Understanding Root Cause for Delay

1. Though patients dread the "life-threatening" aspect, they get caught in prolonged discussions.

2. Patients get advice from many people and often get confused.

Delaying dialysis comes with added issues, as most often patients do not start the right diet for their kidney's condition.

Good pre-dialysis counselling is key to instil confidence in patients and family members. So, it becomes critical to counsel the patients immediately with a good open discussion. Patients need be reassured that this disease can be treated and people can live normally with good dialysis. The option of a kidney transplant as the best treatment must also be explained to the patient. Apart from the doctor, the best person to counsel is another patient who has gone through the treatment successfully.

Some Important Dos and Don'ts

1.   Most of the patients try to fall back on alternate systems in the bargain of avoiding dialysis. What should we do?

      This happens basically out of fear of dialysis. But when another patient shares experiences with dialysis or transplant, this experimentation can be prevented. There is no evidence that for the long term such other alternative treatments are beneficial. In some cases, it has caused adverse results.

2.   What are the common acute complications during dialysis and how can they be avoided?

      •   Catheter-associated infections: It is generally advisable to have a functioning AV fistula during the 1st dialysis itself. If a patient comes as an emergency, then dialysis is started with a catheter that sometimes could get seriously infected. One can prevent infection by talking to the doctor or technician on how to protect the fistula from infection. Also, after starting dialysis, a surgery for AV fistula should be a priority.

      •   Low blood pressure on dialysis: Careful assessment of ideal weight and proper fluid removal is mandatory. Poor weight gain in between dialysis should be avoided by relaxing the salt and water intake. The dialysis technologists should be well-educated and periodic monitoring is needed to see that such precautions are taken.

      •   Breathlessness: Most often, the patient gets breathless due to the uncontrolled intake of salt and water, resulting in high weight gain between 2 dialysis sessions. Uncontrolled blood pressure, severe anaemia and cardiac diseases are other causes. Elderly patients, especially diabetics, should get a cardiac evaluation done prior to dialysis initiation.

3.   What are the likely issues when a person is on long-term dialysis

      •   Vascular access will require periodic review by a vascular surgeon, as the use of the fistula could create narrowing or clot formation. Such issues could be avoided if a person does such check-ups every few years.

      •   Malnutrition – patients should be encouraged to have a high protein diet. Monitoring for albumin monthly and dietitian involvement is key.

- Depression – it is logical to be depressed due to many reasons. Deteriorating health, financial issues, co-morbid medical conditions, lack of family support or they could make a patient feel he/she is a burden to the family. Psychological support would solve some of the issues.

- Hepatitis seroconversion – people on long-term dialysis have a chance to get infected with hepatitis, which can occur due to multiple blood transfusions. Universal precautions in dialysis units and change of tubings are essential. Re-use of tubings must be avoided.

4. Is CAPD –peritoneal dialysis a good alternative?

Diabetics, patients with heart diseases, children who are said to have poor vascular access, aged patients and those who are non-ambulant are ideal candidates for CAPD.

Peritoneal dialysis helps people with greater flexibility to do dialysis while maintaining their jobs/education with lesser restrictions on diet as compared to haemodialysis.

5. Are patients more prone to infections in CAPD?

With improved techniques, the infection rates are significantly lower in CAPD. It has been found that less than 1% out of 48 patients gets infected. Even if there is an infection, in 90% cases it can be safely treated. So, one must feel safe to choose CAPD.

6. Can the dialysis frequency be reduced with time?

The aim of dialysis is to make the patient lead a near-normal life. Good dialysis is important to prevent long-term complications. With good dialysis, there will be an overall improvement in appetite accompanied by maintenance of albumin levels, which ensures good blood pressure control. The doctor advices the number of dialysis needed. Skipping a dialysis could result in excessive fluid accumulation that could be fatal.

7. How much of salt and water can a dialysis patient consume?

Water and salt intake depends on interdialytic weight gain, cardiac status and urine output. Seek your doctor's advice on this as it's critical for good health while on dialysis. A gain of 0.5 to 0.75 kg per day is acceptable. Restriction is recommended for people with high weight gain.

8. How long can a patient lead a normal life on dialysis?

Good dialysis therapy can give you 10 to 15 years of good quality life. CAPD generally works well for 5 years. Then, the patient can switch to haemodialysis. Fortunately, the treatment options – Haemodialysis, CAPD or transplant are interchangeable. A patient who is not doing well on 1 modality can safely be switched to another modality.

Dr. Raju Balasubramaniyam
MBBS, DNB (Gen. Med), DNB (Nephro)
Chief Nephrologist
Kauvery Hospital
Mylapore Chennai

GUIDE TO READ YOUR LAB REPORT

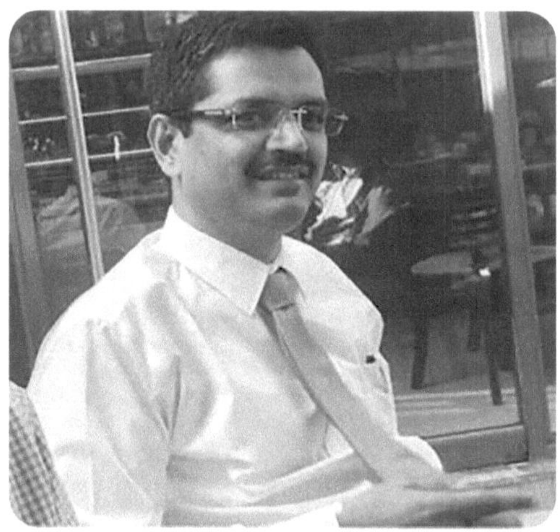

Dr. Manish Mali

If you have chronic kidney disease, you may need some or all of the following tests and measurements:

- Serum Creatinine: Creatinine is a waste product in your blood that comes from muscle activity. It is normally removed from your blood by your kidneys, but when kidney function slows down, the creatinine level rises. Your doctor should use the results of your serum creatinine test to calculate your GFR.

- Glomerular Filtration Rate (GFR): Your GFR tells how much kidney function you have. It may be estimated from your blood level of creatinine. If your GFR falls below 30, you will need to see a kidney disease specialist (called a nephrologist). Your kidney doctor will speak to you about treatments for kidney failure like dialysis or kidney transplant. A GFR below 15 indicates that you need to start 1 of these treatments.

- Blood Urea Nitrogen (BUN): Urea nitrogen is a normal waste product in your blood that comes from the breakdown of protein from the foods you eat and from your body metabolism. It is normally removed from your blood by your kidneys, but when kidney function slows down, the BUN level rises. The BUN can also rise if you eat more protein and it can fall if you eat less protein.

- Urine Protein: When your kidneys are damaged, protein leaks into your urine. A simple test can be done to detect protein in your urine. Persistent protein in the urine is an early sign of chronic kidney disease.

- Microalbuminuria: This is a sensitive test that can detect a small amount of protein in the urine.

- Urine Creatinine: This test estimates the concentration of your urine and helps to give an accurate protein result.

- Protein-to-Creatinine Ratio: This estimates the amount of protein you excrete in your urine in a day and avoids the need to collect a 24-hour sample of your urine.

- Serum Albumin: Albumin is a type of body protein that is made from the protein you eat each day. A low level of albumin in your blood may be caused by not getting enough protein or calories from your diet. A low level of albumin may lead to health problems such as difficulty fighting off infections. Ask your dietician how to get the right amount of protein and calories from your diet.

- nPNA: Your normalised protein nitrogen appearance (nPNA) is a test that may tell if you are eating enough protein. This measurement comes from lab studies that include a urine collection and blood work. Your dietician may ask for an accurate food record to go with this test.

- Subjective Global Assessment (SGA): Your dietician may use SGA to help check for signs of nutrition problems. The dietician will ask you some questions about your daily diet and check your weight and the fat and muscle stores in your face, hands, arms, shoulders and legs. Ask your dietician about your score on the SGA. If your score is too low, ask how to improve it.

- Haemoglobin: Haemoglobin is the part of red blood cells that carries oxygen from your lungs to all parts of your body. Your haemoglobin level tells your doctor if you have anaemia, which makes you feel tired and have little energy. If you have anaemia, you may need treatment with iron supplements and a hormone called erythropoietin (EPO). The goal of anaemia treatment is to reach and maintain a haemoglobin level of at least 11 to 12.

- Haematocrit: Your haematocrit is a measure of the red blood cells your body is making. A low haematocrit can mean you have anaemia and need treatment with iron and EPO. You will feel less tired and have more energy when your haematocrit reaches at least 33 to 36 percent.

- TSAT and Serum Ferritin: Your TSAT (pronounced tee-sat) and serum ferritin (pronounced ferry-tin) are measures of iron in your body. Your TSAT should be above 20% and your serum ferritin should be above 100. This will help you build red blood cells. Your doctor will recommend iron supplements, when needed, to reach your target levels.

- Parathyroid Hormone (PTH): High levels of parathyroid hormone (PTH) may result from a poor balance of calcium and phosphorus in your body. This can cause bone disease. Ask your doctor if your PTH level is in the right range. Your doctor may order a special prescription form of vitamin D to help lower your PTH. Caution: Do not take over-the-counter vitamin D unless ordered by your doctor.

- Calcium: Calcium is a mineral that is important for strong bones. Ask your doctor what your calcium level should be. To help balance the amount of calcium in your blood, your doctor may ask you to take calcium supplements and a special prescription form of vitamin D. Take only the supplements and medications recommended by your doctor.

- Phosphorus: A high phosphorus level can lead to weak bones. Ask your doctor what your phosphorus level should be. If your level is too high, your doctor may ask you to reduce your intake of foods that are high in phosphorus and take a type of medication called a phosphate binder with your meals and snacks.

- Potassium: Potassium is a mineral in your blood that helps your heart and muscles work properly. A potassium level that is too high or too low may weaken muscles and change your heartbeat. Whether you need to change the amount of high- potassium foods in your diet depends on your stage of kidney disease. Ask your doctor what your potassium level should be. Your dietician can help you plan your diet to get the right amount of potassium.

- Body Weight: Maintaining a healthy weight is important to your overall health. If you are losing weight without even trying, you may not be getting the right nutrition to stay healthy. Your dietician can suggest how to safely add extra calories to your diet if needed. On the other hand, if you are slowly gaining too much weight, you may need to reduce calories and increase your activity level. A sudden weight gain can also be a problem. If it is accompanied by swelling, shortness of breath and a rise in blood pressure, it may be a sign of too much fluid in your body. Speak to your doctor if your weight changes noticeably.

- Blood Pressure: Ask your doctor what your blood pressure should be. If your blood pressure is high, make sure to follow all the steps in your prescribed treatment, which may include taking high blood pressure medications, cutting down on the amount of salt in your diet, losing excess weight and following a regular exercise programme.

- Total Cholesterol: Cholesterol is a fat-like substance found in your blood. A high cholesterol level may increase your chance of having heart and circulation problems. For many patients, a good level of total cholesterol is below 200. If your cholesterol level is too high, your doctor may ask you to make some changes in your diet and increase your activity level. In some cases, medications are also used.

- HDL Cholesterol: HDL cholesterol is a type of "good" cholesterol that protects your heart. For many patients, the target level for HDL cholesterol is above 40.

- LDL Cholesterol: LDL cholesterol is a type of "bad" cholesterol. A high LDL level may increase your chance of having heart and circulation problems. For many patients, the target level for LDL cholesterol is below 100. If your LDL level is too high, your doctor may ask you to make some changes in your diet and increase your activity level.

- Triglyceride: Triglyceride is a type of fat found in your blood. A high triglyceride level along with high levels of total and LDL cholesterol may increase your chance of heart and circulation problems.

Dr. Manish Mali
Sr Consultant Nephrologist and Transplant Physician
Aditya Birla Memorial Hospital, Pune, India

PATIENT-CENTRIC ASPECTS

Emotional Challenges of Ckd: Trauma and Need for Support

Early challenges

I recall the first time we left the nephrologist's clinic and we were driving home. All of us were quiet. Different people thinking about different aspects! My son was 15 ½ years old, he had his own teenage worries. As a mother, I was overwhelmed hence, unsure of how to tackle such a sensitive subject. It was far easier to remain silent. But my husband, being a practical person with a scientific mind, used the ride to seek answers. He made a logical assessment of the situation.

Later, at home, he took the discussions to a different level. It began with assessing our son's sad state, emphasising problems likely to be encountered and all the dangers were laid out bare enough to let my stomach churn with fear.

With all the negative aspects of the disease and dangers exposed, he talked about alternative ways of approaching the subject. How to turn the negatives into positives! Even as these evaluations were happening, like a *mother hen* I floated around the house as if I was all-pervading. Truth was, I worried that the teenager was getting so much information that it would terrify him!

But I was wrong.

It worked wonderfully. This was a big lesson I learnt about life. Terror shows reason to fight for life. Some people can pull up their sleeves and get to work, while others may hide under the couch.

In life, we need to make a choice. Get into the battlefield and face the adversary, an eye for an eye. What transpired in our household that day and few days thereafter gave us the courage to go to the battlefield!

The value of logical thinking will be evident in a short while.

Role of a Social Worker/ Counsellor

Any patient leaving a kidney specialist's room comes out in a state of shock. If a few others accompany the person, their reactions are similar. From that moment, subconsciously a certain clock is ticking inside them, spelling death. Irrespective of the person's age and vocation, the patient makes the easy choice.

To drown in self-pity and stop all activity.

To believe their existence is under threat. (Of course, it is, but it needs to be underplayed!)

To wonder about the value of education or staying employed!

And to focus only on healthcare!

During the early days, they have no capacity to plan and determine their future quality of life. For a mind lost in the woods, it has lost its capacity to notice the brightness and warmth of the sun, to wonder about the clear blue sky, to hear the chirping of the birds or see the brilliance of the silver stars in the dark of the night... these are nature's elements that could guide them to safety.

They needed *someone* at that early stage to show compassion with an understanding nod or a gentle touch, to generate a feeling of dependability! Over time, a conversation could build a rapport and draw them into the right approach. They need someone who could show them that contemplating any drastic action should actually be placed right at the bottom of their checklist!

Bringing upfront as *"priority"* should be:

- **Firstly, securing their fort** from all dangers, including being driven by their own erratic mind.

- **Make a plan** for survival.

Ours was something like this:

1. Spent a few hours to understand what had happened! What did we do wrong that landed us in this situation?!

2. Find out as much about the disease as possible.

3. Understood the current stage of the disease and assessed how much time can be considered part of the 'locked up period' before reaching the next stage. Or if we had such knowledge to assess if there is any safe period at all?

4.   What is dialysis? What are the types available? How many people have survived? This topic is painful as death stares you straight in the eyes.

5.   How can we get a transplant? What is the success rate? Who can be medically eligible? What are the transplant laws?

6.   And yes, importantly, the diet!

7.   Finance: Where will funds come from for this treatment?

All the skeletons were now out of the cupboard. On turning it closely to understand all aspects completely, we were drowned in worry as each one looked scarier than the earlier one!

Though number 7 is 'Finance,' placed in the last slot as if to say *money cannot buy everything,* in the case of chronic kidney disease, it ranks ***first.*** Every kidney patient who doesn't have this commodity feels stranded in the middle of a huge deluge. Every rich patient believes he/she can fight CKD with this powerful weapon only to realise that indeed, ***money cannot buy everything!*** Money, money and more money is needed for getting treated and to continue living.

Logical thinking can help you confront your fears and control it. Logic is that guide that leads you to a clear-thinking zone. Death is on the cards for everyone, life is there for people who want and stir in them the *"will"* to survive. The will to survive is very dim but it gathers momentum as you reach another roadblock! One has to tell oneself that it is a delusion and it can be surmounted. One needs to plan how to leap forward.

Back to our way of handling it!

Over the next few weeks, we collected information. My husband made it like a classroom, where both my sons were actively participating. I was in hiding. (As a mother, my sense of guilt was at its peak.) Emotional outbursts were intermittent and my son, who was an exuberant and promising young lad, was now spending more time by himself. At odd times, he was found surfing the Internet for latest information.

But we made a plan that we followed through with many modifications. On top of the chart was the unspoken and spoken agenda! To complete schooling, graduate and be on a career path, so the future has a smoother road moving in some direction.

Research says it all.

Dialysis patients who were jobless or left schooling and education have a high chance of being depressed.

Research says 21% with a job were less depressed.

You can make a choice.

Given above is a sample plan. Make your own survival plan. It can be as exotic as it will be but follow your heart and map your journey to live, with all mental capacities intact.

Airtight plans fail, as we are never sure of the obstacles ahead. But it is also important to break all the walls and to try to penetrate it. Also, never let our fear build its own hillock!

Every person has an individual mental process for handling a serious disease. So, it is important to make your own plan.

Find an Outlet for Your Emotions

Emotional outbursts are a statement of the person's mental state.

Let me say it here now:

It is very much allowed! Go, do it!

It is totally permitted to feel the earth slip from under the feet, to feel ruined and feel that life is at its natural end. There's no need to say I love life and live under a misguided confidence. That could shatter at the 1st resistance it faces.

It's almost as if you were in a tunnel and this huge rock blocked the end, so no light could penetrate it. You have no choice but to sit and quietly work on the rock. Your own patience and persistence will never go unnoticed. Slowly, chips of the rock will fall at your feet when you hit it and apply pressure. When you're frustrated, rest. Give vent to your feelings, but go back to doing the only thing possible. Break the barrier.

The world respects a person who tried hard! People are amazing when it comes to putting you on a pedestal to worship you for your perseverance. Work gets recognised. Courage gets rewarded.

Imagine the total helplessness of a beggar who has only a worn-out shirt, with his pockets empty and with hunger gnawing at him. He can't see any reason to live. It's like he can see no future at all.

That empty feeling is just what chronic kidney disease awakens in you. One feels cheated as if robbed of something precious. So please feel free to express yourself and yell at the world around you. But after that, calm your nerves. Work on making a resolve to survive.

On Facebook, we did a little interaction to understand each person's first reaction to chronic kidney disease. Such a great revelation! So many stood tall through the sands of time, weathering bruises of ego, of body and yet made it to stand testimony of this hour.

Some heart-wrenching observations made are:

Sanjay Nadkarni Said Calmly:

Dazed and confused at 1st to answer your question… Later, devastated, drowned in self-pity, came across an article about a friend, read about his journey, got motivated, picked up my pieces and have been fighting back ever since.

Aditi Ghosh Said Straight from Her Heart:

Shock > denial > anger > bargaining > depression > testing > acceptance

Shaonli Datta Shared Her Experience:

My GP told me over the phone that my creatinine was very high and that I needed to see a nephrologist immediately. I thought, "What is this 'creatinine' and who is a 'nephrologist'?" After a google search, I got a few answers. With fear, I got tested with 3 doctors in 1 month and each time prayed that this was not true. Finally, I accepted it and began my treatment. Took me almost 3 months to accept it, and in those 3 months, the 1ˢᵗ thought I had when I woke up every day was, I was having a bad dream and the thing about the kidney disease has not happened…

Harsh Vardhan Thought about It and Added:

Was shocked at 1ˢᵗ but accepted it as a part of life. But went on research mode… read almost everything on the Internet about chronic kidney disease, about its effects and how it was going to affect my life and if there was any way to reverse it… tried to evade making a fistula for 3 months. Then let my life take its course.

Samiir Halady Spoke Sentimentally about How He Conquered It:

When I was told of the diagnosis, I was stunned. The doctor had tears. I came home and did total silence for 3 days. Only chanting and meditation. After 3 days, I was ready to face anything.

The key is to accept it. It becomes much easier post that.

Ved Prakash Yadav Sounded Doomed as He Said:

When I was 1ˢᵗ introduced to the word 'kidney,' I didn't know what a kidney was. What is it doing in our body? But my father was a little bit aware of it. After seeing his face, I knew that something bad happened to me. After 17 years, I know well what the kidney does. If it fails, you also fail in your life, dreams, future, everything…

Cody Eswaran Spoke of His Struggle with a Lot of Apprehensions:

It was shocking to hear from a visa doctor that my kidneys had failed. Being the 1ˢᵗ time to hear this, I was taken aback. Then, the days passed and doctors changed. Then, I was surprised my creatinine was coming down and going up but good heavens, it didn't cross 4.2. I took a deep breath when I heard people saying that creatinine will never come down as it will gradually increase. After taking medication and proper diet, my creatinine came to 3.2. The next month it moved to 3.5 and then to 3.7, then 3.39. After seeing this, I felt a little relaxed and at the same time, I keep my fingers crossed and hope that I should not go on dialysis at any point. Hope my wish comes true.

Sachin Rao Made a Conclusive Statement:

Marshneil Sinha: My first reaction was, "I've come to the wrong doctor. If I go to the right one, I'll get cured." Only later I realized how little I, or for that matter any average person knew of kidney disease. It took me a lot of time to accept that this was for life. It was not something that gets cured and and gets over and done with.

From all this, clearly, we have something to work on.

1. Talk to your doctor. Get your doubts cleared. Your health is your concern. Doctors have so many patients and are so busy with other serious cases. You have only your case to deal with. Maintain a good rapport with your doctor. While discussing, be a good listener. You will learn many useful things.

2. Talk to your family and friends about your illness. Sharing how you brushed with kidney disease will guide people with hypertension, diabetes, urinary infection or haematuria and proteinuria. You could possibly save them from reaching ESRD.

3. They may ignore you and call you names. You may be scoffed at, but later if your warning was unheeded and they face a similar situation, they will have only their egos to blame.

4. Be your own master in health matters. Search, find information and talk to people at the clinic or dialysis centre. You will learn to accept your situation; maybe yours will be better compared to theirs.

Need for Support

A person who is already facing a health challenge can show some better sense to catch himself/herself before getting into depression. Once this low mental state sets in, help through counsellors must be considered seriously to decrease the impact of 2 major conditions- chronic kidney disease and depression, which could lead to a very grave situation.

Counselling is a help given by qualified people who know how to help people retrace their steps and find the road to survival. However qualified or experienced, you may like to choose someone who can understand you better.

Please do your study before you sign up for counselling. Your friends or physician could guide you on this issue.

Being physically and mentally fit to receive your treatment is important.

Remember this always so you don't miss your opportunity.

All of us are important to our families.

We have to keep our intrinsic values 1 notch higher –

Keep learning skills, try to work and earn and

Smile through life.

No one cares for a loser.

Winner is not one great successful person.

It is one who will stand, head held high,

Not in pride but in humility.

CKD is a great teacher of humility.

Humility brings you honour and with it, bountiful joy!

See that you keep the fire of love around,

Being your kind self.

Diet for Kidney and Life

Be watchful of what you eat based on what you must eat. That's the only way to live. There's no other way. Talk to your doctor and dietician. Their guidance will be of great help. Make your small sacrifices. Leave or limit what is not to be eaten. Better to measure life that is yours and live within the confines. Learn to break those on a rare day – but go back to doing what gave you good health and comfort. CKD is no joke. Learn to live with the knowledge of all essentials.

Exercise

Like diet, exercise is critical for managing all stages of kidney disease. You may discuss with your doctor about what is best suited for your condition. Make a regular schedule for exercise. Thereafter, try to keep to the schedule.

Vasundhara Raghavan

FACEBOOK CHATROOM

To overcome the pain caused by pricks of dialysis needle or being tired of finding money for treatments, people find many diversions and survive. They simply need some comforts to reduce the burden of facing the exhausting disease.

Facebook friends chatted one afternoon. So this was each one diverts attention from CKD.

Jaskiran Sidhu By watching comedy series on television. I am a caregiver of a kidney warrior who amuses himself in this manner.

Sairam Adiraju Reading and sharing knowledge gained in the process with many people so they get some guidance and tips from my own experiences of CKD and kidney transplant.

Harsh Vardhan By reading about history, mythology and politics. I also watch movies and browse the internet.

Vishal Gadhia True amusement for me is sitting silent, reading books and singing devotional songs.

Magda Bonacina Cinema, reading and managing and participating in many renal groups.

Sunanda Brahma True amusement is sitting by the fire on a cold winter evening and sipping a cup of hot aromatic tea.

Shohag Bashar Siddique Take long drives, using gadgets and going to restaurants to understand how they work.

Sangita Shah I am a caretaker. I like to paint, listen to music and drink coffee. My husband, the warrior, amuses himself by watching movies and listening to music.

Navneet Sood Spending time with my wife and daughter, who is an energy powerhouse! I listen to music.... All this make my enjoyable...always.

Kailash Joshi Doing double job to keep busy.

Sweta Bhanawat I amuse myself by cooking food for my family when I am having a good day and of course, online window-shopping.

Jerry Rodrigues Reading and keep myself busy

Gajanan Achintalwar Start the day by reading the newspaper. After a morning walk, some yoga and then hot tea. Watching TV and spending time with my family.

Anjali Uthup Kurian Reading, music, reaching out to people and learning more about renal failure, organ failures and transplant.

Pramod Subramanyam My interests are in playing games, reading, listening to music, watching movies. Most favourite pastime is trying out new variety of dishes.

Deepak Goswami Watching television: news and comedy shows. I love to read, listen to devotional songs in the morning and chat with people on Facebook and in some renal groups.

Merlyn Paul I amuse myself by being with my family and close friends. Surrounded by them, I am constantly reminded that I am blessed and loved.

Sejal Jobanputra This 1 ritual I follow at the start of my day. I say thank you as many times as I can. That gives me so many things to be grateful for and begin the day with happiness.

Sree Devi I am a caretaker for both my warriors, 1 has had a transplant and the other is on dialysis. So, balancing my time between each of them is a task. I keep mind with positive thoughts and listen to devotional songs. I keep hoping all the time.

Praveen Kumar Singh Reading, gardening, playing with my pet dogs, socialising while having my wife around almost all the time. Time flies.

The Kidney Warriors Facebook:

https://www.facebook.com/groups/1569261209995076/

THE RIDE BEYOND REJECTION!

The rhythm of life is determined by so many celestial controls even as our universe makes its own moves or the waves of the sea change their motion.

Whose kidney goes and whose stays results from the throw of a dice.

Many people live with their valuable kidneys for 20, 30, 40 or even 50 years. The dice simply did not select their kidney. Try to tell the aggrieved about this illusive game of dice, it will make sense even if some are more stubborn about their rights. In time, the understanding will surface that not everyone was meant to be a star.

That said, it's very, very difficult to understand the 'why?' and accept it gracefully. To attain a mastery of that philosophy, one has some swallowing to do - of pride and of overwhelming emotion, while letting tears flow freely without any inhibition. The anger and the desperation are an integral part of the game. So, time is needed for the mind to leave the throne and let the heart lead so that kneeling meekly in submission of the superior power is possible.

Life can then be picked up, piece by piece. Surely no one wants to let anyone tread on the scattered pieces of one's self-esteem.

Vasundhara Raghavan

FACING A KIDNEY FAILURE

By Vasundhara Raghavan

Kidney transplants definitely rank higher than dialysis as a treatment, but in spite of much medical advancement, there's a chance of a graft failure.

Research has shown that live donor transplants have better survival rates.

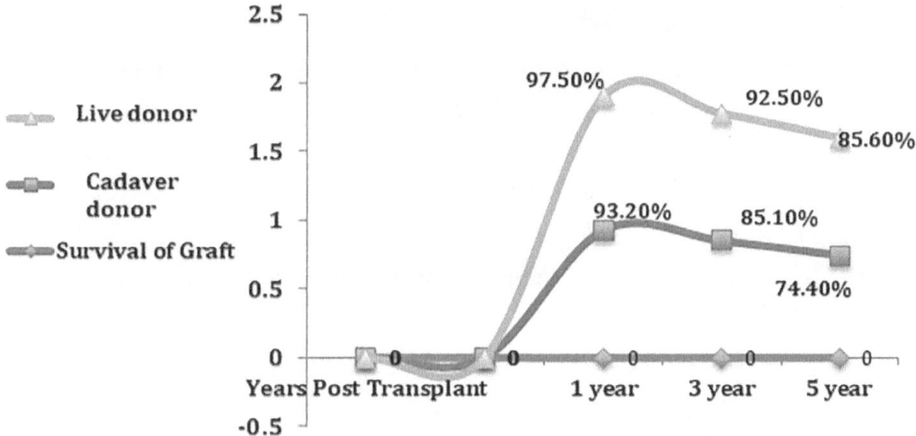

Data used: Kidney Kaplan-Meier Survival Rates for transplants performed 2008-15. Based on OPTN data as of October 20, 2017. Organ Procurement and Transplantation Network, USA. Chart made by Vasundhara Raghavan.

Live or cadaver transplants, many transplants do fail for several reasons:

- Blood clots: if the blood vessels going to the transplanted kidney have clots formed during the surgery, there is a high likelihood the kidney won't receive enough blood supply.

- Infections in the kidney can cause serious complications unless identified and treated early.

- In some cases, though doctors have recommended the organ for transplant, there could be inherent deep-rooted problems in the kidney that could surface after the transplant. Some of them are treatable while some could create problems.

- Early rejections must be promptly attended to. At some point, patient's proactive attention to health care can play a huge role in managing the kidney.

  ✓ You must be alert to catch signs of infections – cold, cough, fever and taking steps to communicate and meet the doctor.

  ✓ Compliance with medications and water intake. Understanding the concept of a kidney transplant and the role of the immunosuppressants is extremely important. These medications suppress the immune system so the body does not attack the kidney. These medications are scheduled. So, one must be conscious of the timings and take them every day to stay ahead in the **graft survival game.**

  ✓ Take simple precautions against infections.

- Acute rejections can be managed with treatments. Though it is more common in the 1st few months, it could happen at any time.

- Chronic rejections mean that the kidney is beyond recovery. The kidney is not accepted by the body and is a long-term problem. The kidney will give up in time.

- Some medications have a tendency of creating problems for the kidney. These could lead to kidney damage.

- In some instances, fluid gets collected around the kidney. If this is not treated in time it can damage the kidney.

- Recurrence of the earlier disease. Some diseases that caused the kidney failure could reoccur.

Most often, the transplant failure is not due to the negligence of the kidney recipient. However, considering how difficult it is to get a transplant, the person must make it a point to:

- Communicate with the nephrologist on small or big issues experienced

- Seek medical advice on changing medication to overcome potentially harmful side effects

- Be always in control of one's health

Rejection Makes Another Life Change

A person who receives a notice, "Your graft has failed!" has to reckon with many aspects of life. However gently this news is delivered, the person's situation cannot be changed. While choosing a transplant, the person has been briefed on survival rates of grafts while subtly conveying the 'cons' of a transplant. But the reality is what determines the future.

The aftermath of a rejection awakens new perceptions of the future. There is:

- **Shock** – how can this happen?

- **Hurt and disappointment** surfaces. Some disappointment that the kidney left them early. No matter that it lasted for 5, 10 or 20 years but their position has now changed.

- **Fear** comes back. Feeling that life is in reverse gear as the person goes back to dialysis. This brings with it a great feeling of insecurity.

- **Acceptance** that they need to start dialysis. Though most people have a transplant after some dialysis treatments, once they experience a transplant they need lots of encouragement to get back on dialysis.

- **Sadness and frustration** to start registration for a transplant once again, if it is possible for them.

- **Abandoned** - During the period that the kidney lasted, people who were strong supporters had moved on in life. There's a new loneliness that envelops them. They need to be showered with love, assurance and understanding. Their file with the transplant team is inactive and they need to find new health support. If the rejection has happened within 90 days of transplant, the transplant team may request for the person's wait time back.

- **Relief** - This is experienced by people whose transplant was a very traumatic experience. They may have faced many serious complications, handling many treatments, effects of side effects and multiple hospitalisations. In such a situation, it may seem better to stay on dialysis.

Apart from the emotional outbursts, in the 1st few months, there is need to relearn many aspects of the disease that they had learnt when 1st diagnosed. This is usually a great challenge.

- Making dietary modifications for haemodialysis

- Getting a fistula in place

- Adapt to rules of the *"water game"*

    ✓ **Dialysis** needs water restriction: 2 litres of fluid split into 2 days

    ✓ **Post-transplant**: Consuming 3-5 litres of water each day post-transplant (as advised by your physician/nephrologist)

    ✓ **Going back on dialysis**: 2 litres of fluid over 2 days

Though dietary changes are also a big issue to contend with, this swing in water consumption is the most dramatic. In hot climates particularly, water restriction is very difficult. Lots of adjustments are needed to be healthy on dialysis, both emotionally and physically.

Good family, friend and community support will steer the person to rise above the constraints and get registered for a transplant or look for another live donor. It is tough, but not impossible.

It is important for the person whose graft has stopped working to realise how important it is to be alive. Shifting focus to other aspects of healthcare and looking for alternate dialysis treatments may help in surviving with great positivity.

GLOSSARY OF TECHNICAL TERMS

Access: Access is created for entering the bloodstream so that dialysis can be done. In the case of haemodialysis, a fistula acts as the access.

Acute coronary syndrome: It involves chest pain and other symptoms when the heart's muscle does not receive enough blood and can cause heart attacks or heart failure.

Acute kidney injury (AKI): AKI is a sudden decline in kidney function. This happens most often due to toxicity of medicines (painkillers and antibiotics), drop in the flow of blood caused by severe infections such as sepsis, dehydration and blockage of urine. It will lead to a build-up of waste products and create an imbalance in electrolytes and body fluids. AKI requires treatment through acute dialysis and is recognised to be associated with greater risk of short-term and long-term death and adverse kidney outcomes.

Albumin is a protein made by the liver. Albumin is found in blood plasma, serum, muscle, the whites of eggs, milk and other animal substances. It is one of the major control mechanisms for blood pressure. A test of blood and urine is done for measuring protein in the blood and urine.

Albuminuria/ Proteinuria: Presence of high albumin or protein in the urine is a sign of some damage to the kidneys. Proteinuria could be the result of long-term hyperglycaemia (high blood sugar levels) of hypertension (high blood pressure).

Anaemia: If a person feels weak, breathless and less energetic, it may be indicative of being anaemic. When blood has a shortage of functioning red blood cells, anaemia occurs. For improvement, iron and erythropoietin will be needed.

Angiotensin-converting-enzyme inhibitors: These are also known as ACE inhibitors. They are medications that widen or dilate your blood vessels to improve the amount of blood your heart pumps and lower blood pressure. By increasing blood flow, ACE inhibitors help to decrease the amount of work your heart has to do. Well-controlled blood pressure by some ACE inhibitors has enabled slow progression in kidney damage in many people with type 2 diabetes.

Artery: A blood vessel that carries blood from the heart to the rest of the body.

Bladder: From the kidney, the urine goes into the organ known as the urinary bladder before being released from the body. Not to be confused with the gallbladder.

Blood cells: The blood is made up of microscopic cells that are known as blood cells. Blood cells consist of red and white cells and platelets.

Blood group: Our blood can be classified into 4 main groups: A, B, AB and O. The classification system is based on hereditary conditions dictating the availability of certain antigens in the cells. Generally, blood and organ donations are based on the match of blood group between the donor and recipient.

Blood pressure: When the blood passes through the arteries, it exerts a certain level of pressure against their walls. This pressure is measured as blood pressure. Blood pressure is an important determinant for many surgeries and indicates the health condition of a person.

American Heart Association redefined high blood pressure in November 2017.

BLOOD PRESSURE CATEGORY	SYSTOLIC mm Hg (upper number)		DIASTOLIC mm Hg (lower number)
Normal	Less than 120	And	Less than 80
Elevated	120-129	And	Less than 80
High blood pressure (hypertension) stage 1	130-139	Or	80-89
High blood pressure (hypertension) stage 2	140 or Higher	Or	90 or Higher
Hypertensive crisis	Higher than 180	And/or	Higher than 120
Note: A diagnosis of high blood pressure must be confirmed by a doctor. Even low blood pressure needs to be evaluated. Data refined and released by American Heart Association in November 2017.			

Body Mass Index (BMI): An individual's weight in kilograms divided by his or her height in metres squared. It is a measurement of body fat.

Bone marrow: In some bones, such as hip and thigh bones, there is a soft tissue in the hollow, interior portion, which is known as bone marrow. New blood cells are formed here.

Cadaveric transplant: This is a transplant surgery done with a kidney or other organs removed from a person who is brain dead or has died in an accident.

Calcium: This is a mineral used in a lot of metabolic processes and also strengthens the bones.

Catheter: A catheter is a flexible plastic tube that is inserted when access to the body's interior is needed.

Cardiovascular: This relates to the heart and the blood vessels involved in blood circulation.

Cholesterol: This is a measure of the level of fat in the bloodstream. There is a risk of having heart diseases or strokes if the blood shows a high cholesterol value. Though high cholesterol is dangerous, the levels can be reduced with a good diet and drugs.

Creatinine: When muscles are used, a waste substance known as creatinine is produced. A blood test is used to measure creatinine and it indicates whether or not the kidney is functioning normally.

The normal values for blood creatinine are: 0.6–1.2 milligrams per decilitre (mg/dl).

Cross-match: The cross-match is different from tissue type or blood group match. Cross-match is a blood test to check for the existence of any antibodies. Antibodies normally help the body fight infections and would react with the donor's kidney. High levels of antibodies may lead to rejection, even if it is a good tissue type match.

Cross-match is done by mixing a sample of the recipient's blood with cells from the donor. If the recipient's blood starts attacking the donor cells, there is the likelihood that the kidney will be rejected.

Dehydration: The body is dehydrated when there is insufficient water in the body for its proper functioning.

Diabetes: When high levels of glucose are found in the blood and urine, a condition popularly known as diabetes is said to be the problem. This happens because of poor functioning of the pancreas. The world over, people with diabetes are at high risk for kidney failure.

Diabetic nephropathy: Kidney disease that results from diabetes. Diabetic nephropathy is the number 1 cause of kidney failure. Almost 1/3rd of people with diabetes develop diabetic nephropathy at some point unless there is strict control of diabetes through medication.

Dialyser: A dialysis machine has a filtering unit known as a dialyser, which removes waste products and excess water from the blood.

Dialysis: The process of removing the waste products and excess water from the blood when the kidneys cease to perform this function properly is known as dialysis.

Dietary acid load (DAL): The body's metabolism produces acids and bases of varying levels based on food consumed. The difference between the acids and bases is called the dietary acid load (DAL) or formally, net endogenous acid production (NEAP). These must be buffered or excreted by the body through respiration or urination in order to maintain an acid-base balance.

Diuretic drugs: Medication administered to increase urine outputs are called diuretics.

Donor: A person who donates an organ, blood or tissue to another person is known as a donor.

Dry weight: The body weight after dialysis is called dry weight. The weight is without excess fluid in the lungs or in the tissues.

Dyslipidaemia: This condition is marked by abnormal concentrations of lipids or lipoproteins such as cholesterol in the blood.

Dysrhythmia: This is an abnormal rhythm, especially a disordered rhythm exhibited in a record of electrical activity of the brain or heart.

Erythropoietin (EPO): When the kidney functions properly, this is a hormone that it produces along with several others. This hormone stimulates the bone marrow to produce red blood cells. But when the kidney fails, the person may become anaemic if lower levels of red blood cells are being produced. In such a situation, EPO injections may be given to perform the hormone's function.

End-stage renal disease (ESRD): When the kidney loses all its functions and reaches the final stage of irreversible loss, it has reached ESRD. Such result may be expected from diabetes, chronic hypertension or glomerulonephritis.

Epidemiology: The study of the distribution and determinants of health-related states or events in specified populations and the application of this study to control health problems.

Expanded criteria donor (ECD): Apart from ideal candidates for organ donation, now people not considered to be ideal or standard are being evaluated as a possible donor. According to these criteria, donors that may be included are people of advanced ages, with previous infection with hepatitis B or hepatitis C, hypertension or diabetes mellitus, abnormal donor organ function and non-heart-beating status of a deceased donor.

Fistula: In order to provide access to the bloodstream for haemodialysis, a vein may be enlarged surgically. This access is called a fistula.

Fluid overload: This is excess water in the body caused by excess consumption of water or not being able to pass enough urine.

Glomerular filtration rate (GFR): Glomerular filtration is the process by which the kidneys filter the blood, removing excess wastes and fluids. To determine the level of the kidney's functioning, a GFR is calculated that shows how well the blood is filtered by the kidneys. This is 1 way to measure remaining kidney function. GFR is usually an estimation, so it is called eGFR. It is derived by using a mathematical formula that is based on a person's size, age, sex and race to compare serum creatinine levels.

GFR: How to Interpret It

Stage	What does that mean?	(GFR level)
At increased risk	Kidneys are at risk due to: diabetes, high blood pressure, family history, old age, ethnic group	More than 90
1	Some damage with normal kidney function	90 or above
2	Damage with mild loss of kidney function	89 to 60
3a	Mild to moderate loss of kidney function	59 to 44
3b	Moderate to severe loss of kidney function	44 to 30
4	Very severe loss of kidney function	29 to 15
5	Kidney failure	Less than 15
GFR number tells you at what level the kidney function remains. Your doctor will tell you the stage of kidney disease. GFR goes down with progression of kidney disease.		

Information source: National Kidney Foundation

Glucose: A sugar found in the blood that is used by cells to produce energy.

Glycaemia: The presence of high blood glucose.

Glycaemic control: For people with diabetes, it is important to maintain glycaemic control. This means to have blood sugar at acceptable levels over a prolonged period of time, usually measured by haemoglobin A1c or fasting blood glucose.

Haemodialysis (HD): A more popular form of dialysis for blood purification. The blood is cleaned outside the body by a dialysis machine, which takes between 3 and 4 hours to finish the process.

Haemoglobin: The red blood cells have haemoglobin, which carries oxygen to all parts of the body.

Haemoglobin A1c (HbA1c) test: This test, also called HbA1c, glycated haemoglobin test or glycohaemoglobin, will determine how well diabetes is being controlled. HbA1c gives an average of blood glucose control over a 6 to 12-week period, which along with periodic home blood glucose monitoring is able to appropriately treat diabetes.

Ideal body weight: An ideal body weight is determined based on the age, sex and height of the person. This is the expected range of people falling within that group.

Immune system: Everybody has an immune system that protects the body from infections and foreign bodies. In the case of a person who has had a transplant, the system is suppressed by medication so that it does not reject the foreign organ. The immune system, therefore, works less effectively.

Immunosuppressant drugs: These are drugs prescribed to transplant patients to make the immune system less effective so that it does not fight the foreign body, which is the transplanted kidney or other organ. Immunosuppressant drugs are required to protect the kidney from being rejected.

Malnutrition: This condition occurs due to lower consumption of food providing protein and energy, usually causing weight loss.

Macroalbuminuria: Albuminuria defined as a relatively high rate of urinary excretion of albumin, which could be greater than 300 milligrams per 24-hour period.

Microalbuminuria: Albuminuria defined as a relatively high rate of urinary excretion of albumin, ranging between 30 milligrams and 300 milligrams per 24-hour period.

Nasogastric tube: This is normally called the NG tube. It is made of a flexible material of rubber or plastic. The tube, used to put substances, including nutrients, into the stomach, is inserted through the nose and then through the oesophagus into the stomach when a patient is unable to eat or drink by mouth. It is normally inserted before a major surgery. Sometimes the tube is used to remove contents from the stomach, including air, small solid objects, fluid and other toxic substances that cannot be removed normally through the stool.

Nephritis: This is an inflammation of the kidneys.

Nephron: The kidney is made up of many small units called nephrons, which do the filtering and balance fluid in the body.

Oedema: This is an abnormal accumulation of water in the body. If the water is accumulated in the lungs, it is called pulmonary oedema.

Omentum: The omentum hangs like a curtain from the bottom of the stomach, right in front of the intestines. It is like a sheet of fatty tissue that stores body fat and it grows as more fat is accumulated. It contains germ-fighting cells that can migrate to the abdomen and helps to seal it off. The omentum, therefore, protects the abdomen from infections. For the surgeon, the omentum acts as a handy tool, something like biological duct tape. Portions of the omentum may be used as a graft in cut areas to heal them. The omentum can also be a source of problems. When its blood supply is interrupted, there are symptoms of severe pain and tenderness that can wrongly be diagnosed as appendicitis.

Peritoneal dialysis (PD): This form of dialysis uses the peritoneum as a filter. The blood is cleaned inside the person's body, not externally as in the case of haemodialysis. PD is a home dialysis programme.

Peritoneum: This is a natural membrane lining the walls of the abdomen.

Peritoneal Cavity: This is the area of the abdomen where the stomach, liver and bowels are found.

Phosphate: An important substance involved with calcium that accumulates when the kidneys fail.

Phosphate binders: In order to avoid the build-up of phosphate in the blood, phosphate binders are prescribed. They absorb excess phosphorus from the blood.

Platelets: These are a type of blood cell that helps in clotting blood.

Polycystic kidney disease: This kidney disease is hereditary and results because of a problem in kidney development. The kidneys get enlarged and are full of sacs filled with fluid, which are known as cysts. This disease sometimes leads to kidney failure.

Potassium: This mineral is normally present in the blood but has to be maintained at a particular level. Higher or lower levels may cause heart problems.

Protein: This is essential for muscle formation. The breakdown products are filtered by the kidney. Meat, fish, dairy products and nuts are rich in protein.

Proteinuria: The presence of excess protein in the urine.

Pulmonary oedema: When the lungs get filled with fluid, the resulting condition is known as pulmonary oedema. It results in breathlessness, especially when lying down flat and exercising.

Pyelonephritis: This is a painless inflammation caused by repeated infections, drugs or other factors. It occurs in the part of the kidneys that is in between filtering units.

Recipient: A person who receives an organ for transplant from a donor.

Rejection: The immune system fights infection and foreign bodies. In the case of a transplant, the organ transplanted is, in fact, a foreign body. The immune system may attack the organ, leading to rejection.

Renal: It is the term used for kidneys. A renal failure means a failure of the kidneys.

Restless legs syndrome (RLS): This neurological disorder causes an individual to experience an uncomfortable sensation in his/her legs leading to an urge to move them. Symptoms occur most often at night, as lying down tends to activate the symptoms. The disorder affects both males and females, with twice as high an incidence in females. With age, this syndrome gets worse.

Satellite haemodialysis unit: A unit that is located away from the main hospital renal unit and provides haemodialysis.

Semi-permeable: A membrane that allows some substances to pass through it.

Serum: The fluid portion of the blood obtained after removal of the fibrin clot and blood cells, distinguished from the plasma in circulating blood.

Serum Creatinine: A product of creatinine phosphate that is filtered from the blood by the kidneys. Serum creatinine levels rise with decreased renal function

Tenckhoff catheter: In a PD, the catheter that allows access to the dialysis fluid to flow in and out from the peritoneal cavity but is capped off when not in use is known as a Tenckhoff.

Tissue type test: A blood test that is conducted to measure the antigens on the surface of the body and its cells.

Transplant: This surgery is done to plant a new organ, which is donated by someone, into a patient who needs it for survival.

Ultra-filtration: This process removes excess water from the blood.

Under dialysis: This happens when dialysis treatment is not sufficient to remove all the water and waste products that are in excess.

Urea: This is 1 of the main waste products that build-up in the blood. In addition to creatinine levels, the levels of urea in the blood are indicative of how the kidneys are functioning.

Uremic seizure: In people who have Acute Kidney Failure or Chronic Kidney Failure, when the GFR drops below 15ml/min it can cause a seizure, which may be mild or severe. It occurs due to build up of toxin and can be a serious condition. Medical attention and advice needed for further action.

Ureters: Urine is carried from the kidneys to the bladder through tubes called ureters.

Urethra: The tube that carries urine from the bladder outside the body.

Urine: This is the fluid produced by the kidneys. It is composed of excess water and the toxic waste products that come from food and are not required by the body.

Urine protein-to-creatinine ratio (UPCR): Ratio of urinary protein to creatinine used to quantify the amount of protein being excreted in urine and used to calculate proteinuria.

Veins: Blood vessels that carry dark-red-coloured blood. They bring impure blood from different parts of the body to the heart for purification. They have less oxygen and are thinner than arteries.

BIBLIOGRAPHY

Listed below are some materials I referenced during the process of writing this book. They helped in my understanding and in providing readers information in simple layman's language. I have attempted to write the book with honesty and as simply as possible.

American Heart Association - www.heart.org/HEARTORG

American Kidney Fund - www.kidneyfund.org

American Urology Association - www.auanet.org

Astellas Transplant - www.transplantexperience.com

Cedar-Sinai Medical Center - www.csmc.edu

Davita - www.davita.com

eMedicineHealth - www.emedicinehealth.com

Healthcommunities.com - www.healthcommunities.com

Kidney School - www.kidneyschool.org

Mayo Clinic - www.mayoclinic.com

MedlinePlus Medical Encyclopedia - www.nlm.nih.gov/medlineplus/encyclopedia.html

MedicineNet.com - www.medicinenet.com

Merriam-Webster Online Dictionary: www.merriam-webster.com

National Kidney Foundation, India - www.nkfi.in

National Kidney Foundation, United States - www.kidney.org

National Kidney Foundation, Southern California - www.kidney.org

National Kidney and Urological Diseases Information Clearinghousekidney.niddk.nih.gov/kudiseases

Nephrology Channel - www.nephrologychannel.com

Texas Pediatric Surgical Associates - www.pedisurg.com

The Kidney Foundation of Canada - www.kidney.ca

University of Iowa Hospitals and Clinics - www.uihealthcare.com

University of Pennsylvania Health System - www.pennmedicine.org

WebMD https://www.webmd.com/

Acharya, V. N., "Status of Renal Transplant in India," *Journal of Postgraduate Medicine* (http://www.jpgmonline.com) 40, no.1 (1994): 158-61.

Stein, Andy, and Wild, Janet, *Kidney Dialysis and Transplants*. London: Class Publishing, 2002.

Garovoy, Marvin R., Guttmann, Ronald D, *Renal Transplantation*. New York: Churchill Livingstone Inc., 1986.

Faris, Michie Hall, *When Your Kidneys Fail*. Southern California: National Kidney Foundation, 1994.

GRATITUDE

To all who came to create a voice for kidney patients. Please know you are not alone.

We are all here, also troubled by disease as you are. We can help you help others, so we teach everyone to lead a better life.

Please Join our Facebook group: The Kidney Warriors https://www.facebook.com/groups/1569261209995076/

Vasundhara Raghavan